OXFORD C

Hyperlipidaemia

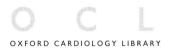

OXFORD CARDIOLOGY LIBRARY

Hyperlipidaemia

Edited by

D. John Betteridge

Professor of Endocrinology and Metabolism
University College London Medical School,
Honorary Consultant Physician,
University College London Hospitals,
London, UK

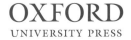

OXFORD
UNIVERSITY PRESS

OXFORD
UNIVERSITY PRESS

Great Clarendon Street, Oxford OX2 6DP

Oxford University Press is a department of the University of Oxford.
It furthers the University's objective of excellence in research, scholarship,
and education by publishing worldwide in

Oxford New York

Auckland Cape Town Dar es Salaam Hong Kong Karachi
Kuala Lumpur Madrid Melbourne Mexico City Nairobi
New Delhi Shanghai Taipei Toronto

With offices in

Argentina Austria Brazil Chile Czech Republic France Greece
Guatemala Hungary Italy Japan Poland Portugal Singapore
South Korea Switzerland Thailand Turkey Ukraine Vietnam

Oxford is a registered trade mark of Oxford University Press
in the UK and in certain other countries

Published in the United States
by Oxford University Press Inc., New York

British Library Cataloguing in Publication Data

Data available

Library of Congress Cataloging in Publication Data

Data available

Typeset by Newgen Imaging Systems (P) Ltd., Chennai, India
Printed in Great Britain by Ashford Colour Press Ltd, Gosport, Hants.

ISBN   978–0–19–954350–2

10 9 8 7 6 5 4 3 2 1

Whilst every effort has been made to ensure that the contents of this book are as
complete, accurate and-up-to-date as possible at the date of writing. Oxford
University Press is not able to give any guarantee or assurance that such is the case.
Readers are urged to take appropriately qualified medical advice in all cases. The
information in this book is intended to be useful to the general reader, but should
not be used as a means of self-diagnosis or for the prescription of medication.

Contents

Preface

It does not seem that long ago when treatment of lipid disorders was the province of a few specialist clinics focusing on severe inherited lipid disorders. Treatment was difficult because there were no well-tolerated, effective and safe drugs and many patients succumbed to premature vascular disease. Clinical trial science now taken for granted was in its infancy and early lipid-lowering trials were inconclusive for a variety of reasons not only due to the ineffectiveness of available drugs but also poor trial design. This situation led to the 'cholesterol controversy' of the early 1990's. It was the introduction of the statin class of drugs to clinical practice which transformed lipid management and importantly enabled definitive clinical trials to be undertaken. The first of these, The Scandinavian Simvastatin Survival Trial reported in 1994, was a landmark trial in many ways: it was of outstanding design with sufficient statistical power such that it has become a paradigm for subsequent clinical trials; it used an effective agent that led to a significant difference in cholesterol concentrations between the placebo and treated groups and its findings of a highly significant reduction in overall mortality helped to stay the 'cholesterol controversy'. Since then many trials have demonstrated benefits of cholesterol-lowering in different patient groups both with and without established cardiovascular disease (CVD). The debate now concerns not so much the ability of drugs to reduce CVD events but the intensity of cholesterol-lowering and at what level of risk intervention is cost-effective.

In this book, experts from Europe address the current state of knowledge starting with the epidemiology background and the role of lipoproteins in atherogenesis. The determination of absolute CVD risk is important in assessing who should be treated, but caveats to this approach are equally important and the diagnosis of important inherited lipid disorders is covered in detail as use of risk charts in these individuals is inappropriate. Secondary causes of hyperlipidaemia are reviewed as it is important for the physician to exclude these conditions and treat appropriately, but in type 2 diabetes dyslipidaemia is an important component of insulin resistance and needs to be addressed in its own right.

Despite the enormous clinical trial data base to inform drug choices, diet and lifestyle remains central and a practical approach to this is provided together with discussion of the various drug classes with particular emphasis on the statins. Despite the general good acceptability of the statins there are situations where knowledge of other drug classes is essential for optimum management, and this is covered in detail. A discussion of combination therapy is provided as this is often needed in more complex lipid disorders. New ways of imaging atheroma are discussed as these techniques are increasingly used in clinical trials and to assess CVD risk beyond conventional risk factors. Finally, there is a chapter on practical management issues.

This book should be of interest to physicians and trainees from many different specialties where CVD risk management is integral to overall patient management. I would like to thank the contributing authors for their excellent chapters and the publishers for their willingness to produce this work.

D. John Betteridge

Contributors

D. John Betteridge
University College London,
London, UK

Rafael Carmena
Universidad de Valencia,
Valencia, Spain

Marie-Therese Coney
The Adelaide & Meath Hospital,
Dublin, Ireland

Ralph D'Agostino
Department of Public Health
Sciences,
Wake Forest University School
of Medicine,
Winston-Salem, NC, USA

Guy De Backer
Gent University Hospital,
Gent, Belgium

Joanna Gouni-Berthold
Department of Internal
Medicine II,
University of Cologne,
Cologne, Germany

Ian M. Graham
Head of Cardiology
The Adelaide & Meath Hospital,
Dublin, Ireland

Julian Halcox
University College
London Hospital,
London, UK

Manish Kalla
University College
London Hospital,
London, UK

Wilhelm Krone
Department of Internal
Medicine II,
University of Cologne,
Cologne, Germany

Tora Leong
The Adelaide & Meath
Hospital,
Dublin, Ireland

Catherine McGorrian
The Adelaide & Meath
Hospital,
Dublin, Ireland

Jonathan Morrell
University College London,
London, UK

Jacqueline Morrell
University College London,
London, UK

José T. Real
Universidad de Valencia,
Valencia, Spain

John Reckless
School for Health,
University of Bath,
Bath, UK

Anton F.H. Stalenhoef
Radboud University Nijmegen
Medical Centre,
Nijmegen, The Netherlands

Anthony S. Wierzbicki
Consultant Chemical
Pathologist, Guy's &
St. Thomas' Hospital London,
London, UK

Abbreviations

ABCA1	ATP-binding cassette A1
ACS	acute coronary syndrome
AFCAPS/ TEXCAPS	Air Force/Texas Coronary Atherosclerosis Prevention Study
ALA	alpha-linolenic acid
AMI	acute myocardial infarction
apo	apolipoprotein
ARH	autosomal recessive hypercholesterolaemia
ASCOT-LLA	Anglo-Scandinavian Cardiac Outcomes Trial Lipid-Lowering Arm
BIP	bezafibrate infarction prevention
BMI	body mass index
CAC	coronary artery calcification
CAD	computer-aided design
CARDS	Collaborative Atorvastatin Diabetes Study
CDP	Coronary Drug Project
CETP	cholesteryl ester transfer protein
CHD	coronary heart disease
cIMT	carotid intimal-medial thickness
CMR	cardiac magnetic resonance
CT	computed tomography
CTT	Cholesterol Treatment Trialists'
CVD	cardiovascular disease
DART	Diet and Reinfarction Trial
DHA	docosahexaenoic acid
DM	diabetes mellitus
EBCT	electron beam CT
EPA	eicosapentaenoic acid
ER	extended-release
FCH	familial combined hyperlipidaemia
FD	familial dysbetalipoproteinaemia
FDB	familial defective apolipoprotein B
FFA	free fatty acids
FH	familial hypercholesterolaemia
FHT	familial hypertriglyceridaemia
FIELD	Fenofibrate Intervention and Event Lowering in Diabetes
FMD	flow-mediated dilation
GI	glycaemic index

HCT	helical CT
HDL	high-density lipoprotein
HDL-C	high-density lipoprotein-cholesterol
HHS	Helsinki Heart Study
HMG-CoA	3-hydoxy-3-methylglutaryl coenzyme A
HPS	Heart Protection Study
HR	hazard ratio
ICER	incremental cost-effective ratio
IDL	intermediate density lipoprotein
IMT	intimal-medial thickness
IR	insulin resistance
IUVS	intravascular ultrasound
JELIS	Japan EPA Lipid Intervention Study
LCAT	lecithin:cholesterol acyltransferase
LDL	low-density lipoprotein
LDL-C	low-density lipoprotein-cholesterol
Lp(a)	lipoprotein(a)
LPL	lipoprotein lipase
LpX	lipoprotein X
LRP	LDL receptor-like protein
MDCT	multidetector CT
MDCTA	MDCT angiography
MI	myocardial infarction
MRI	magnetic resonance imaging
MTP	microsomal triglyceride transfer protein
NCEP	National Cholesterol Education Program
NCEP-ATP III	Third National Cholesterol Education Program Adult Treatment Panel III
NNT	number-needed-to-treat
NPC1L1	Nieman-Pick C1-Like 1
PET	positron emission tomography
PPARα	proliferator-activated receptor α
PROCAM	Prospective Cardiovascular Münster
PROSPER	Prospective Study of Pravastatin in the Elderly at Risk
RCT	randomized clinical trial
RCT	reverse cholesterol transport
RXR	retinoid X receptor
SCORE	Systematic COronary Risk Evaluation
sdLDL	small dense LDL
SEAS	Simvastatin and Ezetimibe in Aortic Stenosis
SHARP	Study of Heart and Renal Protection

SPARCL	Stroke Prevention by Aggressive Reduction in Cholesterol Levels
SR-B1	scavenger receptor class B1
SREBPs	sterol regulatory element binding proteins
TIA	transient ischaemic attack
TLC	therapeutic lifestyle changes
TNT	treat to new targets
VAHIT	Veterans Administration HDL Intervention Trial
VLDL	very low-density lipoprotein
WHO	World Health Organization
WOSCOPS	West of Scotland Coronary Prevention Study

Chapter 1

Epidemiology of cardiovascular disease: the scale of the problem

Guy De Backer

Key points

- The epidemic of cardiovascular disease (CVD) has been and still is very dynamic and heterogeneous when comparing time trends and mortality rates in different places of the world.
- Age-standardized CVD mortality rates have declined in some countries, mainly due to a better management of the essential risk factors.
- Unfavourable trends in CVD incidence are found and foreseen in developing countries due to demographic and to adverse lifestyle changes.
- Comprehensive CVD prevention strategies are needed to promote primary prevention and better implementation of effective preventive actions in patients with established CVD.

1.1 Introduction

The cardiovascular diseases (CVDs) that are discussed in this book are mainly caused by atherosclerosis of the arterial vessel wall. Atherosclerosis is multifactorial in origin and its development is largely related to interactions between genetic and environmental factors. Lipid abnormalities are central to this pathology that underlies clinical entities such as acute myocardial infarction (AMI) or other manifestations of coronary heart disease (CHD), ischaemic stroke, and peripheral artery disease. In this chapter, the scale of the problem of CVD is illustrated from an epidemiological perspective to understand the rationale, the need, and the potential of a comprehensive programme of prevention and management of hyperlipidaemia.

1.2 **CVD: a dynamic epidemic according to mortality statistics**

CVDs have probably always been with us but in the 1950s and 1960s strange changes occurred in CVD mortality statistics in industrialized countries.

It led to alarm signals from the World Health Organization (WHO), such as in 1969 warning the Western world, that we were facing 'mankind's greatest epidemic: CHD has reached enormous proportions striking more and more at younger subjects. It will result in coming years in the greatest epidemic mankind has faced unless we are able to reverse the trend by concentrated research into its cause and prevention'.

Indeed, mortality from CHD had reached high levels and in the 'golden 1960s' Western societies could not afford economic losses due to premature mortality or disability in large numbers of the active workforce.

Suddenly and unexpectedly the picture changed; CHD mortality statistics were levelling off in a few countries in Western Europe and North America followed by other countries (Ford et al. 2007); but the changes were very heterogeneous.

In Figure 1.1, the time trends in age-standardized CHD mortality rates are given from 1968 to 2002 in selected European countries for men.

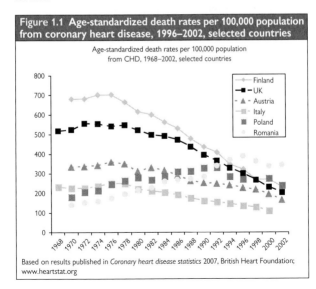

Figure 1.1 Age-standardized death rates per 100,000 population from coronary heart disease, 1996–2002, selected countries

Age-standardized death rates per 100,000 population from CHD, 1968–2002, selected countries

— Finland
— UK
▲ Austria
▦ Italy
■ Poland
Romania

Based on results published in *Coronary heart disease statistics* 2007, British Heart Foundation; www.heartstat.org

Finland had the highest coronary mortality in the world in the late 1960s; this came down to less than half the rate in the most recent years. In the United Kingdom, CHD mortality remained stable for 10yrs and started to decline from the late 1970s onwards (British Heart Foundation 2007).

Austria and Italy had mortality rates less than half that of Finland in 1969; the rates remain comparable for 10yrs but started to decrease from 1980 onwards.

In contrast, Poland and Romania were at the low end of coronary mortality but increased in the 1970s and 1980s; in Poland a reversal took place in 1990, but Romania continued to increase and had in 2002 the highest coronary mortality rate of the six countries presented, while it had the lowest in 1969.

This has resulted in a situation that is not that different from three decades ago in terms of differences between countries; in Figure 1.2, the death rates from CHD are given for men and women, aged 35–74, for the year 1995 or 1996 in selected countries; the rates differ tremendously between nations for both gender.

The age-standardized death rates were higher in women in Latvia and Estonia compared to men in Spain and Portugal, illustrating how relative the protection of women is or how important the effects of the environment.

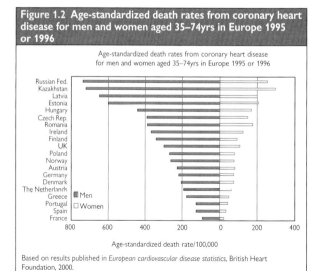

Figure 1.2 Age-standardized death rates from coronary heart disease for men and women aged 35–74yrs in Europe 1995 or 1996

Based on results published in *European cardiovascular disease statistics*, British Heart Foundation, 2000.

Within countries, the changes in CHD mortality rates have also been very different between socio-economic groups. In general, the decline in western countries has been less pronounced in the socially deprived classes. As a result, social differences in CHD have increased over time (Mackenbach et al. 2003).

At the global level, the situation is not more favourable, on the contrary. Demographic changes but also urbanization and unfavourable lifestyle changes are associated with an increase in CVD incidence in most developing countries, not the least in the most populated areas such as India and China (Reddy and Yusuf 1998; Reddy 2004). At this moment, already more than twice as many deaths from CVD occur in developing countries as in developed and in the coming years this will further increase.

The high burden of mortality from CVD in developing countries was estimated at 9 million in 1990 and is expected to increase to 19 million in 2020, compared to an increase from 5 to 6 million in western countries.

In developing countries, the proportion of deaths due to CVD is projected to increase from about 25% in 1990 to more than 40% in 2020.

But there is more to these numbers when they are translated in health care and community costs. In the United States, the annual direct and indirect costs for CHD were 142.5 billion USD in 2006. The economic impact of CVD on health care costs has been estimated at 169 billion Euros in 2003 in the enlarged European Union (Leal et al. 2006). This means an average of 3,724 Euros per capita per year; 62% of this sum is related to direct costs and 21% to productivity losses. The latter number is particularly important for developing countries; indeed, given the demographic composition of these populations and the changes that will take place in the age distribution, not only the increase in CVD is alarming but also the fact that this increase in the coming decades will manifest itself mainly in the economic active part of society. In 1990, 47% of all CVD-related deaths in developing countries occurred before the age of 70 in contrast to only 23% in high-income industrial countries.

Another finding that may seem paradoxical is that in countries where CVD mortality rates have declined, the absolute number of CVD deaths has increased and that CVD remains the major cause of death. This has also to do with demographic changes; the proportion of people aged >65yrs increases in all countries; by preventing premature CVD deaths more people enter into the age classes where a majority of deaths are attributed to CVD. More than 80% of all CVD deaths occur in people over 65. Therefore, the absolute number of CVD deaths increases. Preventive medicine is not aiming at eternal life; its objective is to prevent premature mortality and incapacity;

then the question raises how to define premature death. Given the actual figures of life expectancy in Europe, we may think of CVD death before the age of 75yrs as premature. The scale of the problem of CVD is therefore better illustrated with indicators such as premature mortality or disability-adjusted life years (Murray and Lopez 1996).

In the whole of Europe, the available figures show that CHD, stroke, and other CVD are responsible for 37% of all premature deaths (before the age of 75yrs) in men.

Women are not better off: 43% of all premature deaths are due to CVD.

Considering all DALYs in Europe, the WHO estimated that 27% was related to CVD, 11% to cancer, 20% to neuropsychiatric diseases, and 14% to injuries.

1.3 How well do we explain the dynamics of the CVD epidemic?

For the interpretation of these differences between countries or the different changes over time within populations, it is difficult to differentiate what could be related to a reduced case fatality rate and/or what could be due to primary prevention of clinical events.

Some authors credit the greater use of evidence-based medical therapies such as thrombolysis, percutaneous coronary intervention, aspirin, ACE inhibitors, coronary artery bypass grafting, or statins; others emphasize a better management of the major risk factors such as smoking, arterial hypertension, and dyslipidaemias. To study these questions, different approaches can be used. One of these question was used by the WHO; a global project was set up analysing trends in the incidence of myocardial infarction with trends in risk factor changes and with trends in acute coronary care. This project is known as the MONICA project (Monitoring of trends and determinants of cardiovascular disease) (MONICA 2003).

The MONICA project provided us with the incidence data on coronary event rates, allowing us to compare European countries not only in official mortality statistics but also on the basis of a well-standardized registration of event rates. The average annual event rates illustrated again the large differences that exist in Europe regarding the incidence of this disease. In men, the average annual event rates vary from <200/100,000 in Barcelona to five times this rate (>1,000/100,000) in Finland. In women, the differences are even greater (Müller-Nordhorn et al. 2008).

The first MONICA hypothesis stated that for the population reporting units there is no relationship between 10yrs trend in the major risk factors of serum cholesterol, blood pressure, and cigarette smoking and 10yrs trend in the incidence rates of CHD.

Results show that the variation in trends in coronary event rates was only partially predicted from trends in risk factors. The results showed a modest relation between changes in risk factor score and changes in event rates.

But at any level of change in risk factor score, there was considerable variation in the trends in coronary event rates. The variation in the trends in coronary event rates is incompletely predicted from the trends in risk factors.

The second MONICA hypothesis stated that for the population reporting units there is no relationship between 10yrs trend in case fatality rate and 10yrs trend in acute coronary care. There was a significant association between treatment change and the change in case fatality rate.

Therefore, from the results of the MONICA project it was concluded that both primary prevention and treatment influence mortality trends. The pattern varies in different populations. A high proportion of pre-hospital deaths—mainly sudden cardiac deaths—put great emphasis on primary prevention. Trends are influenced by risk factors. But, the degree to which risk factor changes can explain trends that remain somewhat unclear and incomplete.

Fortunately, as MONICA results showed, quite dramatic reductions in CVD attack rates are possible.

The greatest reduction was by as much as 6.5% per year over a 10-yr period in North Karelia, Finland; this means a reduction of –65% over 10yrs.

The challenge is not merely to predict and to monitor the trends but to influence them. Even modest changes in CVD trends can have a huge public health impact.

Many MONICA centres show that quite substantial changes can take place in 10yrs both up and down. These changes have nothing to do with genetics; they are a result of environmental changes and especially of lifestyle changes. Prevention is possible and it pays off.

Its implementation, however, is not easy and requires not only the health care providers but also the involvement of the whole society. Indeed, in some countries where death rates of CHD were high but now declining—such as in Finland—there is concern about the widening gap in mortality between social classes; the decline in death rates was substantial in all groups but the difference between educational classes—already present in 1970—has increased over time and is much larger in 1990.

Another approach to understand the changes in CVD mortality and incidence rates is by applying models such as the IMPACT CHD policy model developed by a research group in Liverpool.

On the basis of the information on changes in coronary risk factors and on changes in treatment uptake, and using the results from randomized controlled trials with regard to the effectiveness of treatment effects, the model estimates by age and gender the expected influence on CHD mortality.

For instance, between 1981 and 2000, fewer deaths (68,000) from CHD were observed in England and Wales (Unal *et al.* 2005); how well did the model explain that difference?

The model predicted an increase in mortality by worsening of risk factors of 13%, a decline in CHD mortality by improvements in risk factors of 71%; therefore, altogether risk factor changes accounted for a decline of 58%; treatments accounted for another 42%.

Smoking cessation was the greatest contributor to the decline; the worsening was related to obesity, physical inactivity, and diabetes; the gain by treatment was due to a better treatment of AMI, heart failure, and other cardiac conditions.

This model has now been used in different countries and the results are surprisingly similar in most countries with 50–60% of the changes in CHD mortality attributed to changes in risk factors and 40–50% attributed to better treatments, although in Finland more of the decline is related to risk factor changes and less to improvements in therapy.

The model was also applied to Beijing, China, where a rise in CHD mortality was observed from 1984 to 1999; evidence-based medical therapies also have favourable effects in China but this is overruled by the adverse effects of risk factor changes particularly the rise in cholesterol levels (Critchley *et al.* 2004).

Finally, one could quote the results from the INTERHEART study where the large majority of the difference between patients who had suffered an AMI were compared with controls and where population attributable risks of 90% and 94% were observed with a set of 10 risk factors: abnormal lipids, smoking, hypertension, diabetes, abdominal obesity, psychosocial factors, consumption of fruits, vegetables, and alcohol, and regular physical activity accounted for most of the risk of myocardial infarction worldwide in both sexes and at all ages in all regions (Yusuf *et al.* 2004).

1.4 **Conclusions**

- The epidemic of CVD is still very dynamic and heterogeneous both in men and in women; whatever health indicator is used, the actual picture is still challenging; CVD is the leading cause of premature morbidity, a major cause of chronic disability; it causes enormous costs to society

- The decline in CVD mortality in most countries is partially related to less incidence and partially to a reduced lethality which by itself is almost entirely due to less in-hospital deaths in acute conditions and a better prognosis in the chronic phase
- Comprehensive CVD prevention strategies should therefore actively promote primary prevention as well as maximizing the population coverage of effective treatments
- For a better understanding of the recent and future transitions, there is a strong need for comparable and continuous surveillance of CVD, of its risk factors in both the male and the female populations in Europe.

So, there is still ample room for further research in the explanation of the heterogeneity and of the dynamics of the CHD epidemic. On the other hand, we know a lot regarding modifiable risk factors in order to develop preventive strategies that could lessen the burden of premature mortality and disability due to CVD in both genders.

References

British Heart Foundation (2007). Coronary heart disease statistics 2007. Available at www.heartstats.org.

Critchley JA, Liu J, Zhao D, Wei W, and Capewell S (2004). Explaining the increase in coronary heart disease mortality in Beijing between 1984 and 1999. *Circulation*, **110**, 1236–44.

Ford ES, Ajani UA, Croft JB, *et al.* (2007). Explaining the decrease in U.S. deaths from coronary disease, 1980–2000. The *New England Journal of Medicine*, **356**, 2388–98.

Leal J, Luengo-Fernández R, Gray A, Petersen S, and Rayner M (2006). Economic burden of cardiovascular diseases in the enlarged European Union. *European Heart Journal*, **27**, 1610–19.

Mackenbach JP, Bos V, Andersen O, *et al.* (2003). Widening socioeconomic inequalities in mortality in six Western European countries. *International Journal of Epidemiology*, **32**, 830–7.

Marmot M and Elliott P (2005). Coronary heart disease epidemiology: from aetiology to public health. In Marmot M and Elliott P, eds. *Coronary Heart Disease Epidemiology: From Aetiology to Public Health*, 2nd edn, pp. 3–7. Oxford University Press, Oxford, UK.

McGovern PG, Jacobs DR Jr, Shahar E, *et al.* (2001). Trends in acute coronary heart disease mortality, morbidity, and medical care from 1985 through 1997: the Minnesota heart survey. *Circulation*, **104**, 19–24.

MONICA (2003). Monograph and multimedia source book. In Tunstall-Pedoe H, ed. *The World's Largest Study of Heart Disease, Stroke, Risk Factors and Population Trends (1979–2002)*, 244 pp. WHO, Geneva.

Müller-Nordhorn J, Binting S, Roll S, and Willich SN (2008). An update on regional variation in cardiovascular mortality within Europe. *European Heart Journal*, **29**, 1316–26. doi:10.1093/eurheartj/ehm604.

Murray CJL and Lopez AD, eds. (1996). The global burden of disease: a comprehensive assessment of mortality and disability from diseases, injuries and risk factors in 1990 and projected to 2020. Harvard University Press, Cambridge, MA.

Reddy KS (2004). Cardiovascular disease in non-western countries. *The New England Journal of Medicine*, **350**, 2438–40.

Reddy KS and Yusuf S (1998). Emerging epidemic of cardiovascular disease in developing countries. *Circulation*, **97**, 596–601.

Unal B, Critchley J, and Capewell S (2005). Modelling the decline in coronary heart disease deaths in England and Wales, 1981–2000: comparing contributions from primary prevention and secondary prevention. *BMJ*, **331**, 614–19.

Yusuf S, Hawken S, Ounpuu S, on behalf of the INTERHEART Study Investigators (2004). Effect of potentially modifiable risk factors associated with myocardial infarction in 52 countries (the INTERHEART study): case–control study. *The Lancet*, **364**, 937–52.

10

Chapter 2

Lipids, lipoproteins, and atherogenesis

Joanna Gouni-Berthold and Wilhelm Krone

Key points

- Lipids and lipoproteins have a central role in the pathogenesis of atherosclerosis.
- The concentration of low-density lipoprotein (LDL) is strongly and directly related to risk of atherosclerosis whereas high-density lipoprotein (HDL) is inversly related, low HDL being an independent risk factor.
- The role of plasma triglycerides is less well defined.
- The ratio of apolipoprotein B (the major apolipoprotein of LDL) to apolipoprotein A-1 (the major apolipo-protein of HDL) is emerging as the best predictor of atherosclerotic risk.

2.1 Introduction

Arteriosclerosis and its complications remain the major cause of death in developed countries. Cardiovascular diseases (CVDs) cause 38% of all deaths in North America and are the most common cause of death in European men under 65yrs of age (Hansson 2005). Although atherosclerosis has been traditionally viewed as the result of lipid deposition within the vessel wall, recent research has shown that inflammation is also involved in its pathogenesis (Hansson 2005). However, the central role of lipids in the initiation and progression of atherosclerosis remains undisputed.

Cholesterol is absorbed from the intestine and transported to the liver by chylomicrons remnants, which are taken up by the low-density lipoprotein (LDL) receptor-like protein (LRP), Hepatic choles-terol enters the circulation as very low-density lipoprotein (VLDL) and is metabolized through the removal of triglycerides by lipoprotein lipase to remnant lipoproteins and LDL, both of which are subse-quently removed by the LDL receptors. Moreover, the liver has the unique capacity to catabolize cholesterol and convert it into bile salts, which transport cholesterol in the digestive system. Table 2.1 summarizes the composition and roles of the various circulating lipoproteins and apolipoproteins.

Table 2.1 Composition and roles of the various lipoproteins and apolipoproteins [modified from Jain et al. (2007)]

Lipoproteins	Composition	Effect/role
Chylomicrons	95% triglycerides (TG), 5% cholesterol	Mobilize dietary lipids, deliver dietary triglycerides to adipose tissue and muscles, and dietary cholesterol to the liver
VLDL (very low-density lipoproteins)	80% TG, 20% cholesterol	Transport triglycerols to extrahepatic tissues
IDL (intermediate density lipoproteins)	50% TG, 50% cholesterol	Either converted to LDL or taken up by the liver
LDL	10% TG, 90% cholesterol	Principal plasma carrier of cholesterol for delivering to peripheral tissues
HDL (high-density lipoproteins)	5% TG, 95% cholesterol	Increases uptake of cholesterol by the liver
Apolipoproteins (MW [Da])	Lipoprotein association	Comments
Apo A-I (29,016)	Chylomicrons, HDL	Major protein of HDL, activates lecithin: cholesterol acyltransferase (LCAT)
Apo A-II (17,400)	Chylomicrons, HDL	Primarily in HDL, enhances hepatic lipase activity
Apo A-IV (46,000)	Chylomicrons, HDL	Present in triacylglycerol-rich lipoproteins
Apo B-48 (241,000)	Chylomicrons	Found exclusively in chylomicrons, derived from apo B-100 gene by RNA editing in intestinal epithelium; lacks the LDL receptor-binding domain of apo B-100
Apo B-100 (513,000)	VLDL, IDL, LDL	Major protein of LDL, binds to LDL receptor
Apo C-1 (7,600)	Chylomicrons, VLDL, IDL, LDL, HDL	May activate LCAT
Apo C-II (8,916)	Chylomicrons, VLDL, IDL, LDL, HDL	Activates lipoprotein lipase
Apo C-III (8,750)	Chylomicrons, VLDL, IDL, LDL, HDL	Inhibits lipoprotein lipase
Apo D (33,000)	HDL	Associated with LCAT activation
Apo E (34,000)	Chylomicron remnants, VLDL, IDL	Binds to LDL receptor
Apo(a) (300,000–800,000)	LDL	Disulphide bonded to apo B-100, forms a complex with LDL identified as Lp(a)

The earliest form of atherosclerosis, the fatty streak is an accumulation of lipid-laden cells, mostly macrophages, beneath the endothelium. Fatty streaks may later develop to more clinically relevant lesions, the atheromata. These are asymmetric focal thickenings of the intima, consisting of inflammatory and immune cells, vascular endothelial and smooth muscle cells, connective tissue elements, and lipids (Blanco-Colio et al. 2006).

In this chapter, we will discuss the role of LDL-cholesterol (LDL-C) and high-density lipoprotein (HDL)-cholesterol (HDL-C), triglycerides, lipoprotein (a) [Lp(a)], and of the apolipoproteins (apo) B and A-I in the pathogenesis of atherosclerosis.

2.2 LDL-C and atherogenesis

The association of elevated LDL-C levels with atherogenesis has long been established (Murray and Lopez 1997). In patients with hypercholesterolaemia, excess LDL infiltrates the artery wall and is retained in the intima, particularly at the sites of haemodynamic strain. Oxidative and enzymatic modification lead to the release of inflammatory lipids that induce endothelial cells to express leucocyte adhesion molecules. The modified LDL particles are taken up by scavenger receptors of macrophages, which evolve into foam cells (Hansson 2005), the hallmark of atherosclerotic lesions.

LDL-C reduction is now the cornerstone of both primary and secondary prevention of cardiovascular atherosclerotic disease, a fact reflected in the Third National Cholesterol Education Program Adult Treatment Panel III (NCEP-ATP III) guidelines (Grundy et al. 2004), which suggest treatment goals and cut-off LDL-C levels for initiating intervention, summarized in Table 2.2. LDL-C concentrations can be lowered by diet (low in cholesterol and saturated fat), HMG-CoA reductase inhibitors (statins), cholesterol absorption inhibitors, and bile acid binding resins. The most powerful agents for LDL-C lowering are the statins (the various statins available and their doses are summarized in Table 2.3).

Treatment with statins for 5yrs reduces the incidence of major cardiovascular events by about one-fifth per 40mg/dL LDL-C reduction (Baigent et al. 2005). However, approximately 70% of cardiovascular events cannot be avoided in high-risk individuals despite significant LDL-C reduction (Davidson 2005). A probable explanation for this residual risk has been provided recently by the discovery of loss of function mutations in the PCSK9 gene (PCSK9 is an enzyme catalysing the breakdown of LDL receptors), which cause a decrease in LDL-C concentrations by ~40mg/dL and in the prevalence of coronary heart

Table 2.2 ATP III LDL-C goals and cutpoints for therapeutic lifestyle changes (TLC) and drug therapy in different risk categories

Risk category	LDL-C goal	Initial TLC	Consider drug therapy
High risk: CHD* or CHD risk equivalents[†] (10-yr risk >20%)	<100mg/dL (optional <70mg/dL)[‡]	≥100mg/dL	≥100mg/dL[§] (<100mg/dL: consider drug options)[∥]
Moderately high risk: 2+ risk factors** (10-yr risk 10–20%)[††]	<130mg/dL (optional <100mg/dL)	≥130mg/dL	≥130mg/dL (100–129mg/dL: consider drug options)
Moderate risk: 2+ risk factors** (10-yr risk <10%)[††]	<130mg/dL	≥130mg/dL	≥160mg/dL
Lower risk: 0–1 risk factor[‡‡]	<160mg/dL	≥160mg/dL	≥190mg/dL (160–189mg/dL: LDL-lowering drug optional)

* CHD includes history of myocardial infarction, unstable angina, coronary artery procedures (angioplasty or bypass surgery), or evidence of clinically significant myocardial ischaemia.

† CHD equivalents include clinical manifestations of non-coronary forms of atherosclerotic disease (peripheral arterial disease, abdominal aortic aneurysm, and carotid artery disease [transient ischaemic attacks or stroke of carotid origin or >50% obstruction of a carotid artery], diabetes, and 2+ risk factors with 10-yr risk for CHD >20%.

‡ Very high-risk favours the optional LDL-C goal of <70mg/dL, and in patients with high triglycerides, non HDL-C <100mg/dL.

§ If a high-risk person has high triglycerides or low HDL-C, combining a fibrate or nicotinic acid with an LDL-lowering drug can be considered.

∥ When LDL-C lowering drug therapy is employed, it is advised that the intensity of therapy be sufficient to achieve at least a 30–40% reduction in LDL-C levels.

**Risk factors include cigarette smoking, hypertension (BP ≥140/90mmHg or on antihypertensive medication), low HDL-C (<40mg/dL), family history of premature CHD (CHD in male first-degree relative <55yrs of age; CHD in female first-degree relative <65yrs of age), and age (men ≥45yrs; women ≥55yrs).

†† Electronic 10-yr risk calculators are available at www.nhlbi.nih.gov/guidelines/cholesterol.

‡‡ Almost all people with zero or one risk factor have a 10-yr risk <10%, and a 10-yr risk assessment in people with zero or one risk factor is thus not necessary.

Table 2.3 Doses of currently available statins required to attain an approximate 30–40% reduction of LDL-C levels

Drug	Dose (mg/day)	LDL reduction (%)
Atorvastatin	10*	39
Lovastatin	40*	31
Pravastatin	40*	34
Simvastatin	20–40*	35–41
Fluvastatin	40–80	25–35
Rosuvastatin	5–10[†]	39–45

* All of these are available at doses up to 80mg. For every doubling of the dose above standard dose, an approximate 6% decrease in LDL-C levels can be obtained.

† For rosuvastatin, doses available up to 40mg.

disease (CHD) by a remarkable 88% (Cohen *et al.* 2006). Therefore, it appears that for LDL-C lowering, the appropriate cosideration may be not only how low, but also how long (Brown and Goldstein 2006). Further supporting this hypothesis are the results of the 10-yr follow-up of the WOSCOPS primary prevention trial (Ford *et al.* 2007). The study showed that the group originally assigned to pravastatin had better outcomes, even after years of similar statin treatment of the placebo group, suggesting that an early initiation of LDL-C-lowering therapy mitigates the atherosclerotic process.

2.3 HDL and atherogenesis

Multiple epidemiologic studies have established that a low level of HDL-C is an independent risk factor for CVD (Castelli *et al.* 1986). For example, in the Framingham Heart Study, approximately 45% of coronary events occurred in persons with HDL-C levels <40mg/dL (Castelli *et al.* 1986). Furthermore, it has been shown that individuals with HDL-C levels <35mg/dL have an 8-fold higher incidence of CVD compared with those having HDL-C levels >65mg/dL (Castelli *et al.* 1986). About 16–18% of men and 3–6% of women have low levels of HDL (<35mg/dL) (Singh *et al.* 2007). Observational studies have shown that each 1mg/dL decrease in plasma HDL-C concentrations is associated with a 2–3% increased risk of CVD (Gordon and Rifkind 1989). Moreover, each 1mg/dL increase is associated with a 6% lower risk of coronary death, independent from the LDL-C levels (Gordon and Rifkind 1989). Although HDL seems to be protective against CVD, the exact mechanisms of this effect remain unclear. It seems that HDL exerts its antiatherogenic effects through multiple pathways such as reverse cholesterol transport and cholesterol-independent pathways. Reverse cholesterol transport involves the transfer of excess cholesterol from lipid-laden macrophages (foam cells) in peripheral tissues via HDL to the liver, with subsequent excretion of cholesterol into bile or its catabolism. Lipidation of the HDL particles generates nascent (pre-β) HDL. Subsequently, lecithin:cholesterol acyltransferase (LCAT) esterifies free cholesterol within nascent HDL to produce mature α-HDL particles (i.e., HDL$_3$, a smaller more dense particle; and HDL$_2$, a larger less dense particle), which can further take up free cholesterol (Singh *et al.* 2007). Subsequently, the cholesteryl esters in HDL are either taken up by hepatocytes and steroid hormone producing cells or are exchanged for triglycerides in apo B-rich particles through the action of cholesteryl ester transfer protein (CETP). These particles are subsequently taken up by hepatic LDL receptors.

The cholesterol-independent antiatherogenic functions of HDL include antioxidant, anti-inflammatory, and antithrombotic effects (Assmann and Gotto 2004).

Non-pharmacological therapies to increase HDL-C levels include aerobic exercise (5–10%), smoking cessation (5–10%), weight loss (0.35mg/dL per kg of weight lost), moderate alcohol consumption, such as 30–40g/day (i.e., 1–3 drinks) (5–15%), and dietary factors such as n-3 and n-6 polyunsaturated fatty acids (0–5%). Pharmacological therapies include nicotinic acid (increase by 20–30%), statins (5–15%), and fibrates (10–20%). There are many drugs currently tested aimed to increase the levels and/or modify the components of HDL-C such as new nicotinic acid based formulations, cannabinoid-1 receptor antagonists, PPAR agonists, liver X receptor/farnesoid X receptor agonists, and apo A-I and/or phospholipid-derived therapies. High hopes were placed on the CETP inhibitor torcetrapib, which has been shown to decrease carotid atherosclerosis in animals and increase HDL-C levels in humans. However, its development was cancelled in response to the results of four recent trials. First, the Investigation of Lipid Level Management to Understand Its Impact in Atherosclerosis Events (ILLUMINATE) trial (Barter *et al.* 2007) found a 58% increase in all-cause mortality and a 25% increase of cardiovascular events in individuals at high risk for CHD treated with torcetrapib plus atorvastatin compared with those who received placebo plus atorvastatin, even though patients receiving torcetrapib had a 72% increase in HDL-C concentrations. Three other trials that were published the same year also showed no benefits of torcetrapib in atherogenesis, despite similar significant increases in HDL-C levels (Bots *et al.* 2007; Kastelein *et al.* 2007; Nissen *et al.* 2007). The reasons behind these surprising results remain unclear and off-target effects of torcetrapib such as increases in blood pressure and aldosterone levels have been proposed as a possible explanation (Rader 2007; Tall *et al.* 2007). However, these findings stress the point that levels of plasma HDL-C do not predict its functionality and that the focus of research should shift from increasing HDL-C concentrations to improving HDL-C function.

The NCEP-ATP III guidelines (Grundy *et al.* 2004) recognize low HDL (<40mg/dL) as a risk factor for CVD, but no target levels for HDL-C are given.

2.4 **Triglycerides and atherogenesis**

Triglycerides are synthesized *de novo* in the liver where free fatty acids and glycerol are mobilized, packed on to apo B-100, along with cholesterol and phospholipids, and secreted as VLDL. The key enzyme in this assembly process is the microsomal triglyceride transfer protein (MTP), without which apo B would be degraded and VLDL would not be secreted (Le and Walter 2007). The most probable receptor for the uptake of triglycerides is the LRP. A number of plasma enzymes are involved in modulating the lipid constitution of triglycerides in plasma such as CETP, phospholipids transfer protein, lipoprotein lipase, and hepatic triglyceride lipase, the detailed role of which goes beyond the scope of this review.

Even though many studies have demonstrated that elevated triglycerides are associated with CHD risk, a direct association has been questioned because of the inverse association of triglycerides to HDL (McBride 2007). In both the Helsinki Heart Study (Manninen et al. 1992) and the VA-HIT trial (Robins et al. 2001), gemfibrozil treatment achieved significant cardiovascular risk reduction for patients with increased triglyceride levels and low HDL-C levels without significantly lowering LDL. In addition, recent data further strengthen the role of elevated plasma triglycerides in the development of atherosclerosis, especially in women (Bansal et al. 2007; Nordestgaard et al. 2007). An increasing importance is attributed also to the role of non-fasting (2- to 4-hr postprandial) triglyceride concentrations, and their role and use in clinical practice is the subject of active ongoing research.

Interestingly, not all triglyceride-rich lipoproteins are associated with atherosclerosis. For example, for patients with hyperchylomicronemia or type V hypertriglyceridaemia, even with triglyceride levels exceeding 1,000mg/dL, minimal atherosclerotic risk is reported, most probably due to the presence of large, non-atherogenic, lipoprotein particles associated with these disorders (Nordestgaard et al. 2007). Subjects with moderate hypertriglyceridaemia (150–800mg/dL), on the other hand, seem to have high percentages of triglyceride-rich lipoproteins and small dense LDL and HDL particles, all of which are highly atherogenic (McBride 2007).

Given this still disputable causative association between elevated triglycerides and atherosclerosis how should hypertriglyceridaemia be approached in clinical practice? The latest NCEP-ATP III report has no specific recommendations regarding target triglyceride levels. It is introduced as a secondary target of therapy in patients with elevated triglycerides (≥200mg/dL), the non-HDL-C (Grundy et al. 2004), which is the total cholesterol minus HDL-C, a value accurate in non-fasting state and easy to use in everyday practice. Non-HDL-C is considered more predictive of CHD risk than LDL-C levels since it reflects the sum of all atherogenic lipoproteins (Grundy et al. 2004). The non-HDL-C goal is 30mg/dL higher than the LDL-C goal.

Treatment with fibrates is recommended for patients with triglyceride levels over 1,000mg/dL in order to decrease the risk of pancreatitis. After the target levels for LDL-C have been reached,

Table 2.4 Pharmacologic treatment for hypertriglyceridemia				
Drug class	Decrease in TG	Dose	Contraindications	Side effects
Nicotinic acid	17–26%	1,500–2,000mg once a day	Hypersensitivity, hepatic dysfunction	Flushing, pruritus, nausea, hepatitis, migraine
Fibrates	18–45%	Gemfibrozil, 600mg twice a day Fenofibrate, 200mg once a day	Hypersensitivity, hepatic dysfunction, end-stage renal disease	Myositis, cholelithiasis
Statins	5%	Multiple agents	Hypersensitivity, pregnancy, breast-feeding	Myalgia, influenza-like syndrome, weakness, rhabdo myolysis

NCEP-ATP III recommends lowering triglycerides if they are above 200mg/dL (Grundy et al. 2004), although there are no clear data to support this recommendation (Brunzell 2007). Drugs that can be used for the treatment of hypertriglyceridaemia are summarized in Table 2.4 (Brunzell 2007).

2.5 **Apolipoproteins**

Lipoproteins consist of an insoluble lipid core surrounded by a coat of phospholipids, free cholesterol, and apolipoproteins. Each class of lipoprotein particles is associated with specific apolipoproteins (Table 2.1), which stabilize the lipoprotein structure and play an essential role in regulating its metabolism. While some apolipoproteins bind to tissue receptors, others activate or inhibit enzymes modulating metabolic pathways in tissues or in the circulation. In this chapter, we are going to focus on the role of apo B and apo A-I in atherogenesis, since these two are the apolipoproteins most strongly implicated in the pathogenesis of atherosclerosis. Apo A-I and B are structural proteins for HDL and VLDL/LDL, respectively. Apo B-containing lipoproteins carry lipid from the gut and liver to the sites of utilization, while apo A-I-containing particles mediate reverse cholesterol transport, returning excess cholesterol from peripheral tissues to the liver, the only organ capable of excreting cholesterol in significant quantities (in bile) (Marcovina and Packard 2006). Measurement of apolipoprotein levels has methodological advantages over measurement of LDL-C, as it does not require fasting blood samples, is internationally standardized, inexpensive, and may even be conducted on frozen samples.

Apolipoproteins B exists as apo B-48 and apo B-100. Apo B-48 is synthesized in the intestine. There, it is complexed with dietary triglycerides and free cholesterol absorbed from the gut lumen to form chylomicron particles, which in turn are metabolized in the circulation and in the liver. Apo B-100 is synthesized in the liver and is present in VLDL, IDL, and LDL particles (Table 2.1). It is of vital importance for the formation of VLDL, because it interacts with the MTP, a protein that, as previously mentioned, catalyses the transfer of lipids to apo B-100 during the formation of lipoproteins (Akdim et al. 2007). As only one apo B molecule is present in each of these particles, the total apo B concentration reflects the total number of potentially atherogenic lipoproteins (Walldius and Jungner 2004). Apo B-100 is essential for the binding of the LDL receptor, a step necessary for the removal of cholesterol from the circulation.

Apolipoprotein A-I is the major apolipoprotein associated with HDL-C. It also acts as a cofactor for LCAT, an enzyme important for the reverse transport of cholesterol to the liver (Walldius and Jungner 2004). Apo A-I has been shown in various studies to be inversely related to the risk of CHD (Francis and Frohlich 2001; Walldius et al. 2001).

In the Air Force/Texas Coronary Atherosclerosis Prevention Study (AFCAPS/TexCAPS) (Gotto et al. 2000), the ratio of apo B/apo A-I was found to be the best predictor of CHD and in the Apolipoprotein-related Mortality Risk Study (AMORIS) (Walldius et al. 2001), both apo B and the apo B/apo A-I ratio were strongly and positively related to the risk of myocardial infarction. On the basis of this evidence, some support that apo B measurements are a better predictor of CHD than LDL (Walldius and Jungner 2004; Sacks 2006). However, recent studies have pointed out that although the apo B/apo A-I ratio is independently associated with CHD, it adds little to the existing measures of CHD risk assessment (van der Steeg et al. 2007).

Target levels for total apo B concentrations have now been included in a table on the treatment goals of the NCEP-ATP III guidelines who refers to apo B as an alternative (to non-HDL-C) secondary target of therapy when serum triglycerides range from 200mg/dL to 500mg/dL (Grundy 2002). In specific, recommended apo B target levels for subjects with zero to one risk factor are <130mg/dL, for subjects with multiple (2+) risk factors <110mg/dL, and for subjects with CHD or CHD equivalent <90mg/dL. Whether non-HDL-C or total apo B may someday replace LDL-C altogether as the primary target of treatment must depend on the acquisition of enough new data to justify a major conceptual shift in cholesterol management (Grundy 2002).

Currently available drugs that decrease apo B-100 and increase apo A-I concentrations are the statins, nicotinic acid, fibrates, and resins (Walldius and Jungner 2004). Since apo B-100 is the main structural protein present in all atherogenic lipoprotein particles, the inhibition of apo B-100 synthesis in the liver has been suggested as an attractive therapeutic target for the reduction of the concentrations of these lipoproteins. Recent studies using antisense apolipoprotein B-100 nucleotides show a decrease in apo B-100, LDL-C, and triglyceride concentrations, but also an increase in liver-function tests (Akdim et al. 2007). Further clinical trials are under way examining the safety profile and the clinical relevance of these substances.

In summary, the precise role of apolipoproteins as predictors of atherogenesis and their clinical relevance as treatment goals remains to be clarified.

2.6 **Lipoprotein (a)**

Lipoprotein (a), first discovered by Kåre Berg in 1963, consists of a large LDL-like particle to which a large, highly glycosylated apo(a) is linked by a single disulphide bridge. Serum concentrations of Lp(a) vary widely among individuals and are genetically determined to a large extent by the polymorphic apo(a) gene on chromosome 6q27 (Dieplinger et al. 2007). Although the physiological role of Lp(a) is largely unknown, it is a recognized independent risk factor for atherosclerotic CVD (Marcovina and Packard 2006). Lp(a) has been reported to attenuate fibrinolysis and promote coagulation, to activate platelets, to increase the expression of adhesion molecules by endothelial cells, to contribute to foam cell formation, and to be deposited at sites of vascular injury (Tsimikas et al. 2007). However, the exact mechanisms by which this rather enigmatic lipoprotein contributes to atherosclerosis remain unclear.

Data from the study in an Austrian population (Kronenberg et al. 1999) showed that an increase of plasma Lp(a) above the 85th percentile (i.e., plasma levels higher than 32mg/dL) increases the risk for stenosing CHD 4.7-fold and for non-stenosing CHD 1.8-fold. The risk was most pronounced when the LDL-C concentrations were also elevated. Interestingly, elevated Lp(a) levels seem to have different implications to different persons depending, for example, on their race and sex. In this context, Lp(a) seems to confer less risk in blacks than in whites (Sharrett et al. 2001) and in women than in men (Ariyo et al. 2003). Compared with plasma LDL-C, Lp(a) concentrations are relatively resistant to modifications by diet and exercise, as well as to alteration by pharmacological approaches. Nicotinic acid at high doses (4g/day) has been reported to decrease Lp(a) by almost 40% (Carlson 2005). However, the most effective method to decrease

Lp(a) concentrations (by 50% or more) remains the LDL or Lp(a) apheresis, procedures that are costly and laborious (Keller 2007). The most recent workshop on Lp(a) and CVD of the American National Heart, Lung and Blood Institute stated that (1) our understanding of the relative contribution of Lp(a) to the risk burden of CHD is still incomplete and (2) further studies are necessary to examine prospectively the effects of Lp(a) lowering and to identify the mechanism(s) that underlie the pathogenic role of Lp(a) in atherogenesis (Marcovina et al. 2003). At present, Lp(a) is considered an emerging risk factor for atherosclerosis and the treatment goal for Lp(a) concentrations has not been defined.

In summary, while our knowledge of the pathogenesis of atherosclerosis and the role that various lipids and lipoproteins play in it improved significantly over the past years, it still remains incomplete. For example, we still do not know precisely how LDL particles cause the inflammatory and proliferative lesions of the atherosclerotic plaque, and whether the cholesterol content of LDL, which is what we measure, is its most toxic compound or its fatty acids or phospholipids. However, while working on further understanding the mechanisms of atherosclerosis, early and aggressive treatment of elevated cholesterol levels is of utmost importance in order to contain the epidemic of CVD that is ravaging the Western populations over the past decades.

References

Akdim F, Stroes ESG, and Kastelein JJP (2007). Antisense apolipoprotein B therapy: where do we stand? Current Opinion in Lipidology, 18, 397–400.

Ariyo AA, Thach C, Tracy R, and the Cardiovascular Health Study Investigators (2003). Lp(a) lipoprotein, vascular disease, and mortality in the elderly. The New England Journal of Medicine, 349, 2108–15.

Assmann G and Gotto AM (2004). HDL cholesterol and protective factors in atherosclerosis. Circulation, 109, III-8–III-14.

Baigent C, Keech A, Kearney PM, et al. (2005). Efficacy and safety of cholesterol-lowering treatment: prospective meta-analysis of data from 90,056 participants in 14 randomized trials of statins. The Lancet, 366, 1267–78.

Bansal S, Buring JE, Rifai N, Mora S, Sacks FM, and Ridker PM (2007). Fasting compared with nonfasting triglycerides and risk of cardiovascular events in women. JAMA, 298, 309–16.

Barter PJ, Caulfield M, Eriksson M, et al. (2007). Effects of torcetrapib in patients at high risk for coronary events. The New England Journal of Medicine, 357, 2109–22.

Blanco-Colio LM, Martin-Ventura JL, Vivanco F, Michel J-B, Meilhac O, and Egido J (2006). Biology of atherosclerotic plaques: what we are learning from proteomic analysis. Cardiovascular Research, 72, 18–29.

Bots ML, Viseren FL, Evans GW, *et al.* (2007). Torcetrapib and carotid intima-media thickness in mixed dyslipidaemia (RADIANCE 2 study): a randomised, double-blind trial. *The Lancet*, **370**, 153–60.

Brown MS and Goldstein JL (2006). Biomedicine. Lowering LDL—not only how low, but how long? *Science*, **311**, 1721–3.

Brunzell JD (2007). Hypertriglyceridemia. *The New England Journal of Medicine*, **357**, 1009–17.

Carlson LA (2005). Nicotinic acid: the broad-spectrum lipid drug. A 50th anniversary review. *Journal of Internal Medicine*, **258**, 94–114.

Castelli WP, Garrison RJ, Wilson PW, Abbott RD, Kalousdian S, and Kannel WB (1986). Incidence of coronary heart disease and lipoprotein cholesterol levels: the Framingham study. *JAMA*, **256**, 2835–8.

Cohen JC, Boerwinkle E, Mosley TH Jr, and Hobbs HH (2006). Sequence variations in PCSK9, low LDL and protection against coronary heart disease. *The New England Journal of Medicine*, **354**, 1264–72.

Davidson MH (2005). Reducing residual risk for patients on statin therapy: the potential role of combination therapy. *American Journal of Cardiology*, **96**, 3K–13K.

Dieplinger B, Lingenhel A, Baumgartner N, *et al.* (2007). Increased serum lipoprotein (a) concentrations and low molecular weight phenotypes of apolipoprotein (a) are associated with symptomatic peripheral arterial disease. *Clinical Chemistry*, **53**, 1298–1305.

Ford I, Murray H, Packard CJ, Sheperd J, Macfarlane PW, and Cobbe SM (2007). Long-term follow-up of the West of Scotland Coronary Prevention Study Group. *The New England Journal of Medicine*, **357**, 1477–86.

Francis MC and Frohlich JJ (2001). Coronary artery disease in patients at low risk-apolipoprotein A-I as an independent risk factor. *Atherosclerosis*, **155**, 165–70.

Gordon DJ and Rifkind BM (1989). High-density lipoprotein—the clinical implications of recent studies. *The New England Journal of Medicine*, **321**, 1311–16.

Gotto AM Jr, Whitney E, Stein EA, *et al.* (2000). Relation between baseline and on-treatment lipid parameters and first acute major coronary events in the Air Force/Texas Coronary Atherosclerosis Prevention Study (AFCAPS/TexCAPS). *Circulation*, **101**, 477–84.

Grundy SM (2002). Low-density lipoprotein, non-high-density lipoprotein, and apolipoprotein B as targets of lipid-lowering therapy. *Circulation*, **106**, 2526–9.

Grundy SM, Cleeman JI, Bairey-Merz N, *et al.* (2004). Implications of recent clinical trials for the National Cholesterol Education Program Adult Treatment Panel III guidelines. *Arteriosclerosis, Thrombosis, and Vascular Biology*, **24**, e149–61.

Hansson GK (2005). Inflammation, atherosclerosis and coronary artery disease. *The New England Journal of Medicine*, **352**, 1685–95.

Jain KS, Kathiravan MK, Somani RS, and Shishoo CJ (2007). The biology and chemistry of hyperlipidemia. *Bioorganic & Medicinal Chemistry*, **15**, 4674–99.

Kastelein JP, van Leuven SI, Burgess L, *et al.* (2007). Effect of torcetrapib on carotid atherosclerosis in familial hypercholesterolemia. *The New England Journal of Medicine*, **356**, 1620–30.

Keller C (2007). Apheresis in coronary heart disease with elevated Lp(a): a review of Lp(a) as a risk factor and its management. *Therapeutic Apheresis and Dialysis*, **11**, 2–8.

Kronenberg F, Kronenberg MF, Kiechl S, *et al.* (1999). Role of lipoprotein (a) and apolipoprotein (a) phenotype in atherogenesis. Prospective results from the Bruneck study. *Circulation*, **100**, 1154–60.

Le N-A and Walter MF (2007). The role of hypertriglyceridemia in atherosclerosis. *Current Atherosclerosis Reports*, **9**, 110–15.

McBride PE (2007). Triglycerides and risk for coronary heart disease. *JAMA*, **298**, 336–8.

Manninen V, Tenkanen L, Koskinen P, *et al.* (1992). Joint effects of serum triglycerides and LDL cholesterol and HDL cholesterol concentrations on coronary heart disease risk in the Helsinki Heart Study, implications for treatment. *Circulation*, **85**, 37–45.

Marcovina S and Packard CJ (2006). Measurement and meaning of apolipoprotein AI and apolipoprotein B plasma levels. *Journal of Internal Medicine*, **259**, 437–46.

Marcovina SM, Koschinsky ML, Albers JJ, and Skarlatos S (2003). Report of the National Heart, Lung, and Blood Institute workshop on lipoprotein (a) and cardiovascular disease: recent advances and future directions. *Clinical Chemistry*, **49**, 1785–96.

Murray CJ and Lopez AD (1997). Global mortality, disability, and the contribution of risk factors: global burden of disease study. *The Lancet*, **349**, 1436–42.

Nissen SE, Tardif J-C, Nicholls SJ, *et al.* (2007). Effect of torcetrapib on the progression of coronary atherosclerosis. *The New England Journal of Medicine*, **356**, 1304–16.

Nordestgaard BG, Benn M, Schnohr P, and Tybjerg-Hansen A (2007). Nonfasting triglycerides and risk of myocardial infarction, ischemic heart disease, and death in men and women. *JAMA*, **298**, 299–308.

Rader DJ (2007). Illuminating HDL—is it still a viable therapeutic target? *The New England Journal of Medicine*, **357**, 2180–3.

Robins SJ, Collins D, Wittes JT, *et al.* (2001). Relation of gemfibrozil treatment and lipid levels with major coronary events: VA-HIT: a randomized controlled trial. *JAMA*, **285**, 1585–91.

Sacks FM (2006). The apolipoprotein story. *Atherosclerosis Supplements*, **7**, 23–7.

Sharrett AR, Ballantyne CM, Coady SA, *et al.* (2001). Coronary heart disease prediction from lipoprotein cholesterol levels, triglycerides, lipoprotein(a), apolipoproteins A-I and B, and HDL density subfractions: the Atherosclerosis Risk in Communities (ARIC) study. *Circulation*, **104**, 1108–13.

Singh IM, Shishehbor MH, and Ansell BJ (2007). High-density lipoprotein as a therapeutic target: a systematic review. *JAMA*, **298**, 786–98.

Tall AR, Yvan-Charvet L, and Wang N (2007). The failure of torcetrapib: was it the molecule or the mechanism? *Arteriosclerosis, Thrombosis, and Vascular Biology*, **27**, 257–60.

Tsimikas S, Tsironis LD, and Tselepis AD (2007). New insights into the role of lipoprotein(a)-associated lipoprotein-associated phospholipase A2 in atherosclerosis and cardiovascular disease. *Arteriosclerosis, Thrombosis, and Vascular Biology*, **27**, 2094–9.

van der Steeg WA, Boekholdt SM, Stein EA, et al. (2007). Role of apolipoprotein B-apolipoprotein A-I ratio in cardiovascular risk assessment: a case-control analysis in EPIC-Norfolk. *Annals of Internal Medicine*, **146**, 640–8.

Walldius G and Jungner I (2004). Apolipoprotein B and apolipoprotein A-I: risk indicators of coronary heart disease and targets for lipid-modifying therapy. *Journal of Internal Medicine*, **255**, 188–205.

Walldius G, Jungner I, Holme I, Aastveit AH, Kolar W, and Steiner E (2001). High apolipoprotein B, low apolipoprotein A-1, and improvement in the prediction of fatal myocardial infarction (AMORIS study): a prospective study. *The Lancet*, **358**, 2026–33.

Chapter 3

Risk estimation systems in clinical use: SCORE, HeartScore, Framingham, PROCAM, ASSIGN, and QRISK

Catherine McGorrian, Tora Leong, Ralph D'Agostino, Marie-Therese Coney, and Ian M. Graham

Key points

- Atherosclerosis underlying cardiovascular disease (CVD) is a multifactorial disease; hence, global risk estimation is necessary for making clinical decisions.
- Individuals with serious inherited lipid disorders, for example, those with familial hypercholesterolaemia are at high risk and need intensive lipid management and attention to other risk factors.
- Individuals with established CVD have declared themselves to be at high risk and need intensive management.
- For other persons, risk estimation systems described in this chapter help to identify those with unexpectedly high or low risk and hence help to avoid undertreatment or overtreatment.

3.1 Introduction

This chapter is based on a chapter recently written by us (McGorrian *et al.* 2008), but updated and revised to place risk estimation more in the context of hyperlipidaemia.

Since atherosclerosis, and hence cardiovascular disease (CVD), is the product of multiple risk factors, it is clear that a comprehensive evaluation of the combined effects of all major risk factors is the cornerstone of primary prevention. The challenges for the busy health professional are as follows:

- How do I identify people who are at increased risk of a cardiovascular event?
- How do I weight the individual effects of all the causative risk factors, when assessing a person's risk?
- How do I stratify that risk to determine who needs lifestyle advice and who needs additional medical therapy?
- How do I ensure I am not overmedicalizing those persons who are at low risk of an event?

There are two important concepts here, which are stressed by both the American College of Cardiology's 27th Bethesda conference (1996), and the 1994 (Pyorala *et al.* 1994), 1998 (Wood *et al.* 1998), 2003 (De Backer *et al.* 2003), and 2007 (Graham *et al.* 2007) Joint Task Force of European and other Societies on CVD prevention in clinical practice as well as by the US National Cholesterol Education Program (NCEP 2002): the use of a multiple risk factor equation in estimating total risk of a person developing a cardiovascular event, and the need to tailor patient management to overall risk instead of considering single risk factors in isolation.

In the context of hyperlipidaemia, it will be stressed that those with severe hyperlipidaemia, for example, familial hypercholesterolaemia, have declared themselves to be at high risk and to require intensive attention to their lipids and all other risk factors. For other, apparently healthy, people, the use of a risk estimation system can produce surprising results. For example, a 60-yr-old woman with a blood cholesterol level of 8mmol/L (310mg/dL) but no other risk factors has a 2% chance of a fatal CVD event over the next 10yrs. In contrast, a man of the same age with a blood cholesterol level of only 5mmol/L (190mg/dL) may be at 10 times *higher* risk if he is a hypertensive smoker. Who of these examples should receive a statin? On the basis of risk, the man with the cholesterol of 5mmol/L should because of his much higher risk; but available randomized controlled trials do not answer this question. In particular, low-risk women are under-represented.

3.2 **Risk estimation systems**

Cardiovascular risk estimation systems are widely recommended for use in the primary prevention of CVDs. They provide a scientific method for health care professionals to stratify risk, to ensure that those persons at high risk of developing CVDs are identified. Then, appropriate management steps can be undertaken for this group. For the lower risk patients, lifestyle advice is usually appropriate, without recourse to pharmacological therapy.

It should be noted that these risk factor equations are not formulated for use in secondary prevention. Persons with pre-existing CVDs, in particular coronary heart diseases (CHDs), have already identified themselves as being at risk for future events. Therefore, their need for optimum risk factor control is already evident. Furthermore, some subgroups of individuals are also deemed 'high risk' automatically: these include patients with severe, often familial hypercholesterolaemia, with severe hypertension, particularly if target organ damage is present, and with diabetes mellitus. Diabetes is often quoted as being a 'CVD equivalent' (Graham *et al.* 2007), but this is an oversimplification, given the spectrum of diseases ranging from the young, well-controlled type 1 diabetic, to the older type 2 diabetic with other risk factors such as the metabolic syndrome.

It is also important to note that many of these risk equations do not include risk factors such as a family history of premature CHD (which in the Framingham data was found to have an odds ratio for CVD events of 1.3), raised triglyceride levels, or reduced high-density lipoprotein (HDL) cholesterol levels. Neither do many of them have newer risk markers, such as high-sensitivity C-reactive protein. In both Framingham (Wilson *et al.* 1998) and Systematic COronary Risk Evaluation (SCORE) (Conroy *et al.* 2003), caveats are added that features such as the metabolic syndrome and its components will add to total risk, and must be considered when evaluating the results of the risk assessment. Whilst this means that the professional using the scoring system has to keep these caveats in mind, it is probably fair to say that a risk scoring system which included all possible risk factors would be unwieldy to use, and may not be substantially better at identifying high-risk subjects than the existing, simpler scores.

A number of cardiovascular risk estimation systems have been proposed to date, the most well-known being those based on the Framingham function (Wilson *et al.* 1998), which has been used to construct the risk estimation system advised for use by the National Cholesterol Education Program (NCEP) Adult Treatment Panel III (NCEP 2002). The Framingham function also formed the basis of a number of other systems (Haq *et al.* 1995; JBS2 2005). Independent systems include Prospective Cardiovascular Münster (PROCAM) (Assmann *et al.* 2002), the Dundee risk disk (Tunstall-Pedoe 1991), ASSIGN (Woodward *et al.* 2007), QRISK (Hippisley-Cox *et al.* 2007), and a risk estimation system published by Pocock *et al.* (2001). SCORE (Conroy *et al.* 2003) is the European cardiovascular risk estimation tool that is endorsed by the ESC and the Third and Fourth Joint Task Force Recommendations on Cardiovascular Prevention (De Backer *et al.* 2003).

3.3 **Prospective Cardiovascular Münster study**

The investigators in the PROCAM study (Assmann *et al.* 2002) in Europe took a cohort of 5,389 men aged 35–65yrs without an evidence of CVD, and followed them for 10yrs. They used a Cox model to construct a risk algorithm, examining age, low-density lipoprotein (LDL)-cholesterol, smoking, HDL-cholesterol, systolic blood pressure, family history of premature myocardial infarction, diabetes mellitus, and triglyceride levels. The end points were cardiac death or non-fatal myocardial infarction. An integer score was given to each level of risk factor, to give an absolute risk score. Usefully, this score includes such parameters as lipid subfractions and family history. Limitations are the small sample size, that it was based on volunteers rather than a representative population sample, and that no data on women were used in the construction of the initial scoring system. The International Task Force for Prevention of Coronary Heart Disease later published a formula to calculate 10-yr risk of myocardial infarction and sudden cardiac death in women based on PROCAM data (Assmann *et al.* 2002), but as there were only 32 events in 2,810 women, the authors themselves advise using this formula with caution.

3.4 **SCORE and HeartScore**

The SCORE risk estimation system is a very simple graphic representation of the effects of the major risk factors on 10-yr risk of CVD death (Conroy *et al.* 2003; Graham *et al.* 2007). The European Society of Cardiology, the European Atherosclerosis Society, and the European Society of Hypertension originally came together to publish the first Joint Recommendations on the Prevention of Cardiovascular Disease and Clinical Practice in 1994 (Pyorala *et al.* 1994). These recommendations, and the Second Joint Task Force recommendations in 1998 (Wood *et al.* 1998), published a chart to predict 10-yr risk of fatal and non-fatal CHD using age, sex, cholesterol, smoking status, and blood pressure. This chart was based on a risk function, which was derived from the Framingham project.

However, there were some concerns about this approach. Framingham data are from a small, homogenous population in North America, and this was being applied to a large, culturally diverse European population. Second, the end points used in the Framingham data used in these charts included angina pectoris—not an end point that is commonly used in most cohorts, which therefore makes the charts difficult to validate. Third, although the Framingham function has been validated in one study in the United Kingdom (Haq *et al.* 1999), it has also been shown to overpredict risk in a number of

European cohorts (Menotti *et al.* 2000; Hense *et al.* 2003; Marrugat *et al.* 2003). In response to these concerns, and at the request of the ESC, the SCORE investigators developed an independent cardiovascular risk estimation system using European data. Data on 216,000 subjects were pooled from 11 countries in Europe, and mean follow up was 13yrs. Charts were developed for areas with high and low incidences of CVDs (Figure 3.1). They were published in the Third Joint Task Force recommendations, and also in a paper discussing methods (http://www.HeartScore.org). Tables 3.1 and 3.2 show the qualifiers for correct use of the charts.

It is worth considering the end points used in SCORE. Given the heterogeneity of the datasets used, data collection methods could not be standard between the cohorts. Some of the studies only collected follow up data on fatal events. Furthermore, since some of the studies commenced their recruitment and surveys as long ago as the 1970s, the demographics, hospital admission rates, treatment, and even the very definition of end points such as myocardial infarction would have differed significantly from what we see today. Therefore, it was evident that the most appropriate end point was the 'hard' end point of cardiovascular death. This means that, in contrast to the original Framingham end points, and the charts published in the Second Joint Task Force Guidelines, SCORE estimates 10-yr risk of *fatal* cardiovascular events. Therefore, from a 10-yr risk of any cardiovascular event of 20% indicating a subject deemed to be of 'high' cardiovascular risk in the Framingham equation, the emphasis now was on those subjects with a 10-yr risk of a fatal event of 5%. Although this change of end point was a considered one, and was carefully highlighted in the guidelines; it almost inevitably has caused some confusion. Furthermore, some clinicians are uncomfortable with only being able to estimate fatal events, even though a high risk of cardiovascular death would inevitably indicate a higher risk of a non-fatal event. SCORE Plus, a function which estimates total cardiovascular risk, fatal and non-fatal, for high-risk countries, based on FINRISK will be released shortly. Preliminary results suggest that the equivalent of a 5% 10-yr risk of fatal CVD is about 10%, more in younger men and less in women and the elderly.

One problem with all risk charts is that a low absolute risk in a young person may conceal large relative that would mandate intensive lifestyle advice and perhaps drug therapy as the person ages. For this reason, the European Fourth Joint Task Force Recommendations (Graham *et al.* 2007) include a chart that illustrates relative risk (Figure 3.2).

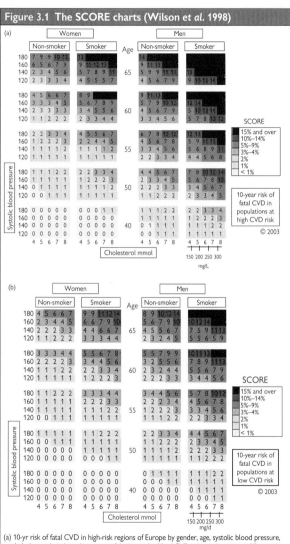

Figure 3.1 The SCORE charts (Wilson et al. 1998)

(a) 10-yr risk of fatal CVD in high-risk regions of Europe by gender, age, systolic blood pressure, total cholesterol, and smoking status. (b) 10-yr risk of fatal CVD in low-risk regions of Europe by gender, age, systolic blood pressure, total cholesterol, and smoking status.

Figure 3.1 is reproduced with permission from the Fourth Joint Task Force of the European Society of Cardiology and other Societies on Cardiovascular Disease Prevention in Clinical Practice (2007). European guidelines on cardiovascular disease prevention in clinical practice: executive summary. *Eur Heart J*, **28**(19): 2375–2414.

Figure 3.2 The SCORE relative risk chart

Systolic Blood Pressure (mmHg)	Non-Smoker: Cholesterol (mmol/L) 4	5	6	7	8	Smoker: Cholesterol (mmol/L) 4	5	6	7	8
180	3	3	4	5	6	6	7	8	10	12
160	2	3	3	4	4	4	5	6	7	8
140	1	2	2	2	3	3	3	4	5	6
120	1	1	1	2	2	2	2	3	3	4

Note: Risk is expressed as a multiple of the lowest risk (one) and not as a precentage.

Table 3.1 Instructions on how to use the charts [From the Fourth Joint Task Force Recommendations (Graham *et al.* 2007)]

- Use the low-risk chart in Belgium, France, Greece, Italy, Luxembourg, Spain, Switzerland, and Portugal; the high-risk chart should be used in all other countries of Europe. (Updated, re-calibrated charts are now available for Belgium, Germany, Greece, the Netherlands, Spain, Sweden, and Poland)
- Find the cell nearest to the person's age, cholesterol, and blood pressure values bearing in mind that risk will be higher as the person approaches the next age, cholesterol, or blood pressure category
- Check the qualifiers
- Establish the total 10-yr risk for fatal CVD

Note that a low cardiovascular risk in a young person may conceal a high relative risk; this may be explained to the person by using the relative risk chart (Figure 3.2). As the person ages, a high relative risk will translate into a high total risk. More intensive lifestyle advice will be needed in such persons

Table 3.2 Qualifiers [From the Fourth Joint Task Force Recommendations Graham et al. 2007)]

- The charts should be used in the light of the clinician's knowledge and judgement, especially with regard to local conditions
- As with all risk estimation systems, risk will be overestimated in countries with a falling CVD mortality rate, and underestimated if it is rising
- At any given age, risk appears lower for women than for men. This is misleading since, ultimately, more women than men die from CVD. Inspection of the charts shows that their risk is merely deferred for 10yrs
- Risk may be higher than indicated in the chart in:
    - Sedentary and obese subjects, especially those with central obesity
    - Those with a strong family history of premature CVD
    - The socially deprived
    - Subjects with diabetes risk may be 5-fold higher in women and 3-fold higher in men compared with those without diabetes
    - Those with low HDL cholesterol or high triglycerides
    - Asymptomatic subjects with evidence of preclinical atherosclerosis, for example, a reduced ankle-brachial index or on imaging such as carotid ultrasonography or CT scanning

Figure 3.2 is reproduced with permission from the Fourth Joint Task Force of the European Society of Cardiology and Other Societies on Cardiovascular Disease Prevention in Clinical Practice. (2007). European guidelines on cardiovascular disease prevention in clinical practice: an executive summary. *Eur Heart J*, **28**(19):2375–2414.

One strength of the SCORE system is that it is paper-based, and the risk levels are read directly off it. There is no calculation required on the part of the clinician. Furthermore, it is free to disseminate without copyright. This is highly advantageous when it comes to making the charts available in the public forum. The downside of this paper chart, however, is that other risk factors cannot be added without generating an unwieldy portfolio of multiple charts. The potential solution to this is the electronic version of SCORE, HeartScore (http://www.HeartScore.org). This web-based tool is based on the SCORE function, and allows for country-specific recalibration using national mortality data. To date, country-specific risk estimation systems have been published for Belgium, Germany, Greece, The Netherlands, Poland, Spain, and Sweden with others in production or pending publication. Forthcoming projects seek to include other risk factors such as HDL cholesterol, body mass index, and family history of CVD.

The first version of HeartScore was based on the Danish PRECARD™ computer-based risk estimation and management system, as developed by Thomsen et al. (2001). HeartScore is based on the SCORE function, and uses the same risk factors and algorithims. It is available through the European Society of Cardiology website (www.escardio.org), and high risk, low risk, and country-specific versions are available. Once the risk factors for a particular patient are inputted, absolute risk at current and ideal risk factor levels are displayed, and these graphs can be printed and given to the patient for his or her own reference (Figure 3.3). Details inputted on a particular patient can also be saved under the doctor's personal login code, and referred to during future consultations.

Score and HeartScore also provide risk factor management advice, and tailor it to the level of total risk estimated. There are also management strategies described for situations when individual risk factors are markedly elevated. HeartScore, in particular, is geared towards the provision of management advice, as links lead to pages with advice taken from the Pocket Guidelines of the Fourth Joint Task Force. This is acknowledged to be a particular strength of the program. Given that best risk factor management changes as more evidence is published, there are clear benefits to this adaptable web-based system.

In addition, in response to requests from countries in which clinicians do not always have ready access to broadband in their day to day practises, a standalone, desktop version of HeartScore is currently in test phase and due for release in 2008.

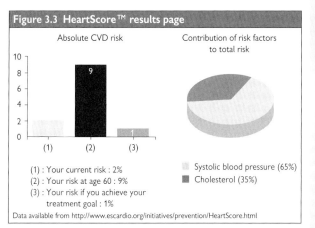

Figure 3.3 HeartScore™ results page

Absolute CVD risk

Contribution of risk factors
to total risk

(1) : Your current risk : 2%
(2) : Your risk at age 60 : 9%
(3) : Your risk if you achieve your
treatment goal : 1%

Systolic blood pressure (65%)
Cholesterol (35%)

Data available from http://www.escardio.org/initiatives/prevention/HeartScore.html

3.5 **The Framingham study**

The Framingham study is a classic prospective epidemiological cohort
study. It began in 1948 when 5,209 residents aged 28–62 in the town
of Framingham, Massachusetts, were enrolled, and subsequently
reassessed with surveys every 2yrs. From 1971 onwards, 5,124 of the
original cohort's offspring and offspring's spouses were enrolled
(Kannel *et al.* 1979). More recently, a third generation cohort has
been added. Prior to Framingham, the prevailing concept was that a
single cause of CVD would be found. However, this of course was
not found to be the case; rather, a number of predisposing 'risk factors' were identified (Kannel *et al.* 1961), including increasing age,
male gender, hypertension, high serum cholesterol, and LDL subfraction, low HDL cholesterol, cigarette smoking, glucose intolerance
and diabetes mellitus, obesity, physical inactivity, and left ventricular
hypertrophy. It is no exaggeration to say that the Framingham study
has fundamentally shaped our understanding of both the aetiology of
atherosclerotic CVDs and their prevention.

In 1973, the Framingham investigators published CHD risk equations (American Heart Association 1973). In 1991, this risk system
was updated using data from both the original Framingham cohort
and the Framingham Offspring cohort (Anderson *et al.* 1991).
It included the data on those persons aged 30–74, who were free
of stroke, transient ischaemic attack, heart failure, intermittent

claudication, and CHD (angina pectoris, coronary insufficiency, myocardial infarction, and sudden death) at the beginning of the study. A Cox proportional hazards model was used, and a chart was devised where each risk factor is given weighting in points, including age, sex, total cholesterol, HDL cholesterol, systolic and diastolic blood pressure, diabetes, smoking status, and left ventricular hypertrophy on ECG. From the summary of these points, the absolute 5-yr and 10-yr CHD risk can be calculated, and this can then be compared to the baseline risk in the community (Figure 3.4).

However, the end points used in this 1991 risk equation included the 'soft' end point of angina pectoris, which is not commonly used as an end point in other studies. Therefore, an updated coronary prediction model was published in 1998 (Wilson *et al.* 1998), this allowed the calculation of the risk of 'hard' CHD end points only and of 'hard' and 'soft' end points (including angina pectoris). For the most recent National Cholesterol Education Program Adult Treatment Panel III guidelines (NCEP 2002), the NCEP have updated the Framingham risk score to use only 'hard' end points (Figure 3.5). They recommend the use of this equation for risk estimation in primary prevention in persons with more than two risk factors, and 'high risk' individuals are deemed to be those with a 10-yr risk of CHD events of >20%. The NCEP have a web-based risk calculator at http://www.nhlbi.nih.gov/guidelines/cholesterol/. Also available from the NCEP guidelines are summaries of specific management advice for those persons at high risk, including an 'At-a-glance' desk reference.

The most recent Framingham risk estimation function was published in 2008 (Woodward *et al.* 2007). This estimates the 10-yr risk of a first cardiovascular event. Cardiovascular events include fatal and non-fatal: myocardial infarction, coronary insufficiency, angina, ischaemic or haemorrhagic stroke, transient cerebral ischaemia, heart failure, and intermittent claudication. The 10-yr risk can be calculated using a simple points scoring sheet. Sex-specific baseline survivals and beta coefficients for the risk factors have been used. The function preformed well both in terms of discrimination (C-statistic 0.763 in men to 0.793 in women) and calibration. They have also presented a risk Function, which includes only non-laboratory-based measures that are routinely measured in primary care: age, body mass index, systolic blood pressure, antihypertensive medication use, current smoking, and diabetes status. Multipliers for the calculation of risk of specific CVD end points are also given.

Figure 3.4 Framingham-based coronary disease risk prediction score sheet

1. Find points for each risk factor

Age (if female) (yr)				Age (if male) (yr)				HDL cholesterol			
Age	Points	Age	Points	Age	Points	Age	Points	HDL	Points	HDL	Points
30	−12	41	1	30	−2	48–49	9	25–26	7	67–73	−4
31	−11	42–43	2	31	−1	50–51	10	27–29	6	74–80	−5
32	−9	44	3	32–33	0	52–54	11	30–32	5	81–87	−6
33	−8	45–46	4	34	1	55–56	12	33–35	4	88–96	−7
34	−6	47–48	5	35–36	2	57–59	13	36–38	3		
35	−5	49–50	6	37–38	3	60–61	14	39–42	2		
36	−4	51–52	7	39	4	62–64	15	43–46	1		
37	−3	53–55	8	40–41	5	65–67	16	47–50	0		
38	−2	56–60	9	42–43	6	68–70	17	51–55	−1		
39	−1	61–67	10	44–45	7	71–73	18	56–60	−2		
40	0	68–74	11	46–47	8	74	19	61–66	−3		

Total cholesterol (mg/dl)		Systolic blood pressure (mm Hg)					
Chol	Points	SBP	Points	SBP	Points		
139–151	−3	98–104	−2	150–160	4		
152–166	−2	105–112	−1	161–172	5		
167–182	−1	113–120	0	173–185	6		
183–199	0	121–129	1				
200–219	1	130–139	2				
220–239	2						
240–262	3						
263–288	4						
289–315	5						
316–330	6						

Other factors	Points	
	Yes	No
Cigarette smoking	4	0
Diabetes		
Male	3	0
Female	6	0
ECG-LVH	9	0

Figure 3.4 (Cont.)

2. Add points for all risk factors

(Age) + (Total chol) + (HDL) + (SBP) + (Smoking) + (Diabetes) + (ECG-LVH) = (Total)

Note: Minus points subtract from total.

3. Look up risk corresponding to point total

Points	Probability (%) 5yr	10yr	Points	Probability (%) 5yr	10yr	Points	Probability (%) 5yr	10yr	Points	Probability (%) 5yr	10yr
≤1	<1	<2	9	2	5	17	6	13	25	14	27
2	1	2	10	2	6	18	7	14	26	16	29
3	1	2	11	3	6	19	8	16	27	17	31
4	1	2	12	3	7	20	8	18	28	19	33
5	1	3	13	3	8	21	9	19	29	20	36
6	1	3	14	4	9	22	11	21	30	22	38
7	1	4	15	5	10	23	12	23	31	24	40
8	2	4	16	5	12	24	13	25	32	25	42

4. Compare with average 10-year risk

Age (yr)	Probability (%) Women	Men	Age (yr)	Probability (%) Women	Men	Age (yr)	Probability (%) Women	Men
30–34	<1	3	45–49	5	10	60–64	13	21
35–39	<1	5	50–54	8	14	65–69	9	30
40–44	2	6	55–59	12	16	70–74	12	24

HDL, high density lipoprotein; SBP, systolic blood pressure; ECG-LVH, left ventricular hypertrophy by electrocardiography.

Based on the 1998 risk tables (National Cholestrol Education Program 2002) and available from http://www.nhlbi.nih.gov/about/framingham/index.html

Figure 3.5a Framingham-based coronary risk score for 'hard' end points, from the National Cholesterol Education Program guidelines (De Backer et al. 2003)

Table III.1–6. 10-Year Risk Estimates for Women (Framingham Point Scores)

Age	Points
20–34	−7
35–39	−3
40–44	0
45–49	3
50–54	6
55–59	8
60–64	10
65–69	12
70–74	14
75–79	16

Total cholesterol	Points at Ages 20–39	Points at Ages 40–49	Points at Ages 50–59	Points at Ages 60–69	Points at Ages 70–79
<160	0	0	0	0	0
160–199	4	3	2	1	1
200–239	8	6	4	2	1
240–279	11	8	5	3	2
≥280	13	10	7	4	2

	Points at Ages 20–39	Points at Ages 40–49	Points at Ages 50–59	Points at Ages 60–69	Points at Ages 70–79
Nonsmoker	0	0	0	0	0
Smoker	9	7	4	2	1

HDL	Points
≥60	−1
50–59	0
40–49	1
<40	2

Systolic BP	If Untreated	If Treated
<120	0	0
120–129	1	3
130–139	2	4
	3	5
≥160	4	6

Point Total	10-Year Risk	Point Total	10-Year Risk
<9	<1%	20	11%
9	1%	21	14%
10	1%	22	17%
11	1%	23	22%
12	1%	24	27%
13	2%	≥25	≥30%
14	2%		
15	3%		
16	4%		
17	5%		
18	6%		
19	8%		

From Third Report of the Expert Panel on Detection, Evaluation, and Treatment of High Blood Cholesterol in Adults (ATP III Final Report), NIH Publication No. Ø2-5215, National Cholesterol Education Program, National Heart, Lung, and Blood Institute, National Institutes of Health, September 2002. The Framingham study data were also used in the development of the Joint British Societies' risk assessment charts. These are published in the most recent JBS2 guidelines (Haq et al. 1995), and an electronic form is also available at http://www.bnf.org/BNF/extra/current/450024.html

The Framingham study data were also used in the development of the Joint British Societies risk assessment charts. These are published in the most recent JBS2 guidelines (2005), and an electronic form is also available at http://www.bnf.org/.

Figure 3.5b Framingham-based coronary risk score for 'hard' end points, from the National Cholesterol Education Program guidelines (De Backer et al. 2003)

Table III–5. Estimate of 10-Year Risk for Men (Framingham Point Scores)

Age	Points
20–34	−9
35–39	−4
40–44	0
45–49	3
50–54	6
55–59	8
60–64	10
65–69	11
70–74	12
75–79	13

Total Cholesterol	Points at Ages 20–39	Points at Ages 40–49	Points at Ages 50–59	Points at Ages 60–69	Points at Ages 70–79
<160	0	0	0	0	0
160–199	4	3	2	1	0
200–239	7	5	3	1	0
240–279	9	6	4	2	1
≥280	11	8	5	3	1

	Points at Ages 20–39	Points at Ages 40–49	Points at Ages 50–59	Points at Ages 60–69	Points at Ages 70–79
Nonsmoker	0	0	0	0	0
Smoker	8	5	3	1	1

HDL	Points
≥60	−1
50–59	0
40–49	1
<40	2

Systolic BP	If Untreated	If Treated
<120	0	0
120–129	0	1
130–139	1	2
140–159	1	2
≥160	2	3

Point Total	10-Year Risk	Point Total	10-Year Risk
<0	<1%	11	8%
0	1%	12	10%
1	1%	13	12%
2	1%	14	16%
3	1%	15	20%
4	1%	16	25%
5	2%	≥17	≥30%
6	2%		
7	3%		
8	4%		
9	5%		
10	6%		

From Third Report of the Expert Panel on Detection, Evaluation, and Treatment of High Blood Cholesterol in Adults (ATP III Final Report), NIH Publication No. Ø2-5215, National Cholesterol Education Program, National Heart, Lung, and Blood Institute, National Institutes of Health, September 2002. The Framingham study data were also used in the development of the Joint British Societies' risk assessment charts. These are published in the most recent JBS2 guidelines (Haq et al. 1995), and an electronic form is also available at http://www.bnf.org/

3.6 ASSIGN and QRISK

Recently, two other cardiovascular risk estimation systems were introduced: ASSIGN (Assessing cardiovascular risk using SIGN guidelines to ASSIGN preventive treatment) (Woodward et al. 2007) in Scotland and QRISK (Hippisley-Cox et al. 2007) in England. Both include two additional risk factors: family history and an area measure of social deprivation. ASSIGN was derived using the SHHEC

(Scottish Heart Health Extended Cohort) study; a cohort study containing 6,419 men and 6,618 and is available on the Internet (www.assign-score.com). QRISK was derived from a large dataset, containing pooled medical records from 318 UK general practices, including 1.28 million patients (Hippisley-Cox *et al.* 2007). The authors have demonstrated better discrimination and calibration compared to the original Framingham function; however, there are some problems with the methodology of this risk function, including the use of imputed lipid measures for 70% of the participants and the use of data from general practice registers as opposed to prospective population studies. While the inclusion of social deprivation as a risk factor is important, because both scores use area measures of deprivation based on postal code these risk scores may be difficult to apply to other populations.

3.7 **Conclusion**

While severely hyperlipidaemic subjects and those with established CVD need immediate and intense risk factor management, most asymptomatic persons will require assessment of their total risk to facilitate a logical risk management plan. Currently available risk estimation systems aim to assist the busy physician to assess total risk easily and quickly. All available systems have strengths and weaknesses. Electronic systems that interact with prevention guidelines continue to evolve.

References

27th Bethesda Conference (1996). Matching the intensity of risk factor management with with the hazard for coronary disease events. *Journal of American College of Cardiology*, **27**, 957–1047.

American Heart Association (1973). *Coronary Risk Handbook: Estimating the Risk of Coronary Heart Disease in Daily Practice*. American Heart Association, Dallas, TX.

Anderson KM, Wilson PWF, Odell PM, and Kannel WB (1991). An updated coronary risk profile. *Circulation*, **83**, 356–62.

Assmann G, Cullen P, and Schulte H (2002). Simple scoring scheme for calculating the risk of acute coronary events based on the 10 year follow-up of the prospective cardiovascular Munster (PROCAM) study. *Circulation*, **105**, 310–15.

Conroy RM, Pyorala K, Fitzgerald AP, *et al.* (2003). Estimation of ten-year risk of fatal cardiovascular disease in Europe: the SCORE project. *European Heart Journal*, **24**, 987–1003.

D'Agostino RB Sr, Vasan RS, Pencina MJ, *et al.* (2008). General cardiovascular risk profile for use in primary care: the Framingham Heart Study. *Circulation*, **117**, 743–53.

De Backer G, Ambrosioni E, Borch-Johnsen K, et al. (2003). Third Joint task force of European and other Societies on Cardiovascular disease prevention in clinical practice. European Guidelines on cardiovascular disease prevention in clinical practice. *European Heart Journal*, **24**, 1601–10.

Graham I, Atar D, Borch-Johnsen K, et al. (2007). European Guidelines on Cardiovascular Disease Prevention in Clinical Practice. *European Journal of Cardiovascular and Prevention and Rehabilitation*, **14**(Suppl 2), 2375–414.

Haq IU, Jackson PR, Yeo WW, and Ramsay LE (1995). Sheffield risk and treatment table for cholesterol lowering for primary prevention of coronary heart disease. *The Lancet*, **346**, 1467–71.

Haq IU, Ramsay LE, Yeo WW, Jackson PR, and Wallis EJ (1999). Is the Framingham risk function valid for northern European populations? A comparison of methods for estimating absolute coronary risk in high risk men. *Heart (British Cardiac Society)*, **81**, 40–6.

Hense HW, Schulte H, Lowel H, Assmann G, and Keil U (2003). Framingham risk function overestimates risk of coronary heart disease in men and women from Germany—results from the MONICA Augsburg and the PROCAM cohorts. *European Heart Journal*, **24**, 937–45.

Hippisley-Cox J, Coupland C, Vinogradova Y, Robson J, May M, and Brindle P (2007). Derivation and validation of QRISK, a new cardiovascular disease risk score for the United Kingdom: prospective open cohort study. *BMJ*, **335**, 136–47.

JBS2 (2005). Joint British Societies' guidelines on prevention of cardiovascular disease in clinical practice. British Cardiac Society, British Hyperlipidaemia Association, British Hypertension Society, British Diabetic Association. *Heart*, **91**, 1–52.

Kannel WB, Dawber TR, Kagan A, et al. (1961). Factors of risk in the development of coronary artery disease—six-year follow up experience; the Framingham study. *Annals of Internal Medicine*, **55**, 33–50.

Kannel WB, Feinleib M, McNamara PM, Garrison RJ, and Castelli WP (1979). An investigation of coronary heart disease in families: the Framingham Offspring Study. *American Journal of Epidemiology*, **110**, 281–90.

Marrugat J, D'Agostino R, Sullivan L, et al. (2003). An adaptation of the Framingham coronary heart disease risk function to European Mediterranean areas. *Journal of Epidemiology & Community Health*, **57**, 634–8.

McGorrian C, Leong T, D'Agostino RB Sr, and Graham I (2008). Risk estimation systems in clinical use: SCORE, HeartScore and the Framingham system. In *Therapeutic Strategies in Cardiovascular Risk*, Chapter 11, pp. 159–71. Atlas Medical Publishing Ltd.

Menotti A, Puddu PE, and Lanti M (2000). Comparison of the Framingham Risk function-based coronary chart with risk function from an Italian population study. *European Heart Journal*, **21**, 365–70.

NCEP (National Cholesterol Education Program) (2002). Expert panel on detection, evaluation and treatment of high blood cholesterol in adults (Adult treatment panel III) final report. *Circulation*, **106**, 3143–421.

Pocock SJ, McCormack V, Gueyffier F, Boutitie F, Fagard RH, and Boissel JP, on behalf of the INDANA Project Steering Committee (2001). A score for predicting risk of death from cardiovascular disease in adults with raised blood pressure, based on individual patients' data from randomised controlled trials. *BMJ*, **323**, 78–81.

Pyorala K, DeBacker G, Graham I, *et al.* (1994). Prevention of coronary heart disease in clinical practice: recommendations of the Second Joint Task Force of European Society of Cardiology, European Atherosclerosis Society and European Society of Hypertension. *Atherosclerosis*, **110**, 121–61.

Thomsen TF, Davidsen M, Jorgensen HIT, Jensen G, and Borch-Johnsen K (2001). A new method for CHD prediction and prevention based on regional risk scores and randomized clinical trials; PRECARD and the Copenhagen Risk Score. *Journal of Cardiovascular Risk*, **8**, 291–7.

Tunstall-Pedoe H (1991). The Dundee Risk Disc for management of change in risk factors. *European Heart Journal*, **303**, 744–7.

Wilson PW, D'Agostino RB, Levy D, Belanger AM, Silbershatz H, and Kannel WB (1998). Prediction of coronary heart disease using risk factor categories. *Circulation*, **97**, 1837–47.

Wood D, DeBacker G, Faergeman O, Graham I, Mancia G, and Pyorala K (1998). Prevention of coronary heart disease in clinical practice: recommendations of the Task Force of the European and other Societies on Coronary Prevention. *European Heart Journal*, **19**, 1434–503.

Woodward M, Brindle P, and Tunstall-Pedoe H, for the SIGN group on risk estimation (2007). Adding social deprivation and family history to cardiovascular risk assessment: the ASSIGN score from the Scottish Heart Health Extended Cohort (SHHEC). *Heart*, **93**, 172–6.

Chapter 4

Primary dyslipidaemias

Anton F. H. Stalenhoef

> ## Key points
>
> - Primary hyperlipidaemias are autosomal dominant or recessive inherited disturbances in lipid metabolism, which become manifest either from early childhood or later in life.
> - Clinical manifestations are premature ischaemic vascular disease, xanthomatosis and other lipid depositions in the body, and acute pancreatitis.
> - The molecular defect is explained by mutations in genes, which encode proteins that play a major role in the formation, secretion, transport, or uptake of lipoproteins.
> - The most common forms of primary dyslipidaemias are multifactorial heterogeneous disorders with several genetic, metabolic, and environmental factors interacting and contributing to the clinical phenotype.
> - Family investigation is usually crucial for proper diagnosis and case finding of persons at risk for vascular disease.

4.1 Introduction

Understanding the underlying pathophysiology of the primary dyslipidaemias is important for several reasons: (1) to get insight in the process of atherosclerosis, because dyslipidaemias are causally related to the development of ischaemic vascular disease; (2) to develop proper treatment of these disorders and prevent early atherosclerosis; and (3) to prevent and treat other clinical sequelae such as disfiguring xanthomata and life-threatening acute pancreatitis.

This chapter deals with the common forms of primary dyslipidaemia as well as rare genetic disorders in lipoprotein metabolism and describes briefly the genetic background, the clinical symptoms, and pathophysiology. These rare genetic disorders have been instrumental for our understanding of both normal lipid physiology and the process of atherosclerosis in humans. Although enormous progress has been made in the understanding of the molecular mechanisms underlying these 'simple' monogenetic diseases, it is also becoming increasingly clear that by interaction with other genes and/or environment there is a wide variation in the phenotypical or clinical expression of these disorders.

The dyslipidaemias can be distinguished schematically in disturbances in the formation, transport, or metabolism of (1) triglyceride-rich lipoproteins [very low-density lipoproteins (VLDL) and chylomicrons], (2) cholesterol-rich lipoproteins [intermediate density lipoproteins (IDL) and LDL], and (3) high-density lipoproteins (HDL). It should be clear that this arrangement is rather artificial because the lipoproteins interact extensively in the circulation and exchange components from both their surface and core; alterations in the composition of secreted VLDL particles will influence the composition and thereby metabolic pathways of both LDL and HDL.

4.2 **Familial hypercholesterolaemia**

Familial hypercholesterolaemia (FH) is an autosomal dominant inherited lipid disorder caused by one of the many (>1,000) mutations in the gene for the LDL receptor, leading to increased total and LDL-cholesterol levels (two times elevated compared to matched controls) from early childhood, and later on in life to typical tendon xanthomata and premature atherosclerosis (Figures 4.1 and 4.2). The lack of functional receptors for LDL on the liver cell surface causes a delayed clearance of LDL from plasma. The clinical expression varies widely and is influenced by other risk factors for cardiovascular disease (Austin *et al.* 2004; Brunzell 2007). The disorder occurs in 1 out of 400–500 individuals in most western countries, but in certain areas in the world, the incidence is much higher due to a founder effect. Homozygous patients with two mutated LDL-receptor alleles (total serum cholesterol four times elevated) develop xanthomata (including skin xanthomata) and atherosclerosis at very young age. Untreated they usually die before the age of 20–30yrs due to complications of vascular disease and aortic valvular stenosis.

Similarly, mutations in the gene coding for apolipoprotein (apo) B also reduce LDL clearance, resulting in the disorder familial defective apolipoprotein B (FDB), which is clinically indistinguishable from FH (Rader and Hobbs 2005).

Recently, it was demonstrated that seemingly non-functional variants in exons and introns of the LDL-receptor gene can effect the normal transcription of these genes and RNA splicing by the disruption or generation of splice sites and branch points, also leading to severe hypercholesterolaemia (Bourbon *et al.* 2007).

Figure 4.1 Xanthomata of extensor tendons of the hands in familial hypercholesterolaemia

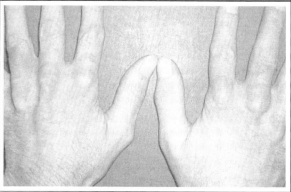

Figure 4.2 Achilles tendon in familial hypercholesterolaemia (note surgery scar)

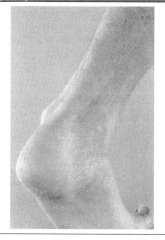

In addition to common mutations in the LDL receptor and apoB genes, a few rare mutations in genes involved in cholesterol metabolism also cause the FH clinical phenotype: mutations in the proprotein convertase subtilisin/kexin type 9 (*PCSK9*) gene encoding for neural apoptosis-regulated convertase 1 (NARC-1), of which the mechanism behind the hypercholesterolaemia is still unknown; and mutations in the autosomal recessive hypercholesterolaemia (ARH) gene, which encodes an adaptor protein that is necessary for endocytosis of the LDL-receptor/LDL complex (Rader et al. 2003).

The clinical phenotype caused by mutations in LDL-receptor, ApoB, or PCSK9, and characterized by elevated levels of plasma LDL-cholesterol is nowadays referred to as autosomal dominant hypercholesterolaemia. See also Table 4.1.

4.3 Familial combined hyperlipidaemia

Familial combined hyperlipidaemia (FCH) is the most common heritable lipid disorder, affecting 1–2% of the general population and up to 20% of the survivors of a premature myocardial infarction. The lipid profile of FCH is characterized by elevated levels of VLDL and/or LDL and apo B. Furthermore, decreased levels of HDL-cholesterol and the presence of small dense LDL (sdLDL) are typical features. The phenotype becomes fully apparent only after the second decade of life. There are no special clinical features besides premature cardiovascular disease (CVD). Patients with FCH are often obese and insulin resistant and share several characteristics with subjects who are diagnosed with the metabolic syndrome.

FCH was first described based on the level of plasma total cholesterol and/or triglycerides above the 90th percentile adjusted for age and gender, within a family with multiple types of hyperlipidaemia and the presence of premature CVD. The disorder was therefore also named 'multiple type hyperlipidaemia'. A major problem in the diagnosis of FCH is that the pattern of hyperlipidaemia may vary over time also within one individual, leading to a non-consistent diagnosis of FCH. A nomogram developed from follow-up studies of a large cohort of FCH families, based on plasma total cholesterol and triglycerides levels, adjusted for age and gender, and absolute apo B levels appears to predict the diagnosis of FCH best in a particular patient (Veerkamp et al. 2004).

4.3.1 Pathogenesis of FCH

FCH is thought to be caused by hepatic overproduction of VLDL-apo B, either with or without impaired clearance of VLDL from plasma, leading to the different FCH lipid phenotypes. The most important determinant of increased VLDL-apo B production is most likely

Table 4.1 Primary dyslipoproteinaemias

Name	Plasma lipids (mmol/L)	Elevated lipoprotein fraction	Cause	Estimated prevalence in population
Familial hypercholesterolaemia (FH):				
Heterozygous	TC = 7–13	LDL	LDL receptor defect	1:400–500
Homozygous	TC >13			1:106
Familial defective Apo B-100 (FDB)	TC = 7–13	LDL	Apo B mutation	1:1,000
FH3	TC = 7–13	LDL	PCSK9-mutation	<1 in 2,500
Familial dysbeta-lipoproteinaemia (FD)	TC = 7–13	VLDL/chylo-micron remnants	ApoE mutation and increased	1:5,000
	TG = 4–8	(β-VLDL)	VLDL secretion	
Familial combined hyperlipidaemia (FCH)	TC = 6–9 TG = 3–8	LDL and/or VLDL	Elevated production	1:200–300
			VLDL-apo B	
Familial hypertri-glyceridaemia (FHT)	TG = 3–9	VLDL (+chylo microns)	Impaired clearance/increased production VLDL–TG	1:500

increased concentrations of plasma free fatty acids. Visceral obesity and insulin resistance may play an important role in the pathogenesis of FCH, but do not fully explain elevated levels of apo B, which supports the concept of separate, genetic determinants in the aetiology of FCH (de Graaf et al. 2002).

4.3.2 The genetic origin of familial combined hyperlipidaemia

The complex genetics of FCH is still not fully understood. Originally, FCH was thought to be a homogeneous single-gene disorder with a major effect on triglyceride levels and a secondary effect on cholesterol levels. Segregation analyses, however, have implicated major genes in FCH that control triglycerides levels, apo B levels, sdLDL, and insulin resistance (Juo et al. 1998). Several linkage analyses have been performed in various FCH study populations, resulting in the identification of multiple loci for FCH. One locus, on chromosome 1q21-23, has been identified as a major locus for FCH in Finnish FCH families and has subsequently been replicated in several other FCH study populations. Another repeatedly identified locus for FCH is located on chromosome 11q, a region including the apolipoprotein A1/C3/A4/A5 gene cluster. Furthermore, loci on several other chromosomes have been identified. So far, this has not led to the identification of major genes that fully explain the molecular basis of FCH. Several candidate genes have been shown to modify the phenotypic expression of FCH in certain families (upstream stimulatory factor 1 (USF1), apolipoprotein A1/C3/A4/A5) (Lee et al. 2006; van der Vleuten et al. 2007).

Furthermore, environmental factors, such as diet, exercise, and smoking, are known to play a role in the clinical presentation of FCH. So, at present FCH is known as a multifactorial heterogeneous disorder with numerous genetic, metabolic, and environmental factors contributing to its complex phenotype.

4.4 Familial hypertriglyceridaemia

Familial hypertriglyceridaemia (FHT) is a heritable lipid disorder, which also comes fully manifest at adult age. It is inherited in an autosomal dominant fashion. Its prevalence is estimated to 1 in 500 subjects in the population. It is usually caused by an overproduction of large triglycerides-rich lipoproteins by the liver in combination with a delayed clearance of triglycerides from plasma (Stalenhoef et al. 1986). The level of triglycerides varies from slightly increased to strongly elevated. The concentration of LDL-cholesterol is normal to low and HDL-cholesterol is decreased. Additional environmental factors [high fat diet, overweight, medication (oestrogens), excess alcohol consumption, uncontrolled type 2 diabetes mellitus] can aggrevate the dyslipidaemia and lead to grossly elevated triglycerides levels (>50mmol/L), which becomes visible as lipaemic plasma due to the scattering of light by the presence of large chylomicron and VLDL particles (Figure 4.3). This can be accompanied by eruptive xanthomata on the trunk and extremities and carries a high risk for acute pancreatitis. This is also the case in patients with rare autosomal recessive disorders in triglyceride metabolism, who are homozygous for mutations in the genes that encode for the enzyme LPL or its cofactor apo C-II (see below). By limitation of fat intake and treatment of possible underlying disorders, the lipaemia and xanthomata can disappear within a few days to weeks (Figure 4.4).

Figure 4.3 Eruptive xanthomata in severe hypertriglyceridaemia

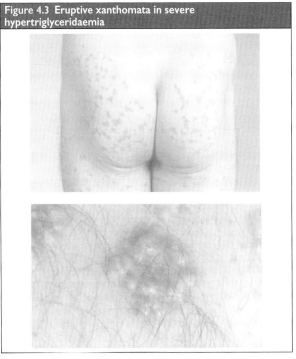

Figure 4.4 Tubero-eruptive xanthomata familial dysbetalipoproteinaemia (type III hyperlipoproteineaemia)

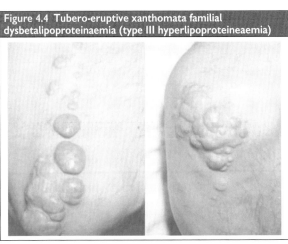

The underlying molecular and genetic defect in FHT is not fully understood, as is the case with FCH, and many additional environmental and metabolic factors also play a role in the expression of this disorder. FHT could well be arranged among the broad spectrum of FCH, whereby in the case of FHT oversecretion and delayed clearance of large triglycerides-rich particles are more pronounced than hepatic overproduction of apo B.

4.5 **Familial dysbetalipoproteinaemia**

Familial dysbetalipoproteinaemia (FD), also known as type III hyperlipidaemia and remnant removal disease, is a relatively rare, autosomal recessive inherited disorder of lipid metabolism, characterized by strongly elevated plasma levels of cholesterol and triglycerides (Mahley and Rall 1995). It occurs in a frequency of around 1 in 5,000 individuals, becomes fully expressed at adult age in men and only even after menopause in women, due to the protective effect of oestrogens. The dyslipidaemia is caused by an accumulation in plasma of remnants of chylomicrons and VLDL (also known as β-VLDL). This fraction is abnormally rich in cholesterol [VLDL-cholesterol to plasma triglyceride ratio >0.69 (on a mmol/L base)]. The presence of homozygosity for a particular isoform of apolipoprotein E, E2, which serves as a ligand for hepatic receptors, is necessary for the development of this disorder. Apo E2 is the mutant apolipoprotein that differs from the wild-type apo E (apo E-3) by a single amino acid substitution (arginine replaced by cysteine at residue 158). The presence of this genotype results in a delayed clearance of the catalytic remnants of chylomicrons and VLDL after lipolysis by LPL, due to insufficient binding of these remnants to their hepatic receptors. However, hyperlipidaemia and subsequently vascular disease become only manifest in combination with overproduction of these lipoproteins by the liver, which occurs in uncontrolled diabetes mellitus, hypothyroidism, subjects with FCH, excess alcohol intake, or obesity. The prevalence of the homozygous apo E2/2 genotype is around 1% in the population; of these subjects, only a few per cent become hyperlipidaemic. This lipid disorder is clinically characterized by tubero-eruptive xanthomata, yellow palmar streaks (Figure 4.5), and premature coronary and peripheral vascular disease (intermittent claudication). The dyslipidaemia is usually very responsive to treatment. Next to the common autosomal recessive form of FD, several kindreds have been described with dominant forms of FD, in which the affected subjects are heterozygous for a particular apo E variant [apo E-Leiden, apo E2 (Lys146→Gln]. Dominant FD arises early in life without distinction between men and women.

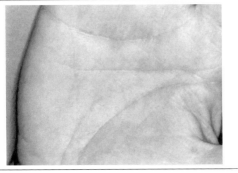

Figure 4.5 Palmar streaks in familial dysbetalipoproteinaemia (type III hyperlipoproteineaemia)

4.6 Familial HDL deficiency

Familial HDL deficiency, also called familial hypoalphalipoproteinaemia, is defined as a plasma HDL-cholesterol level below the 10th percentile, whereas LDL-cholesterol and triglyceride levels are normal, without apparent secondary causes of low plasma HDL-cholesterol (Rader and Hobbs 2005). The condition is usually inherited in an autosomal dominant fashion. The metabolic aetiology of this disease is mostly unknown; the low HDL levels appear to be primarily due to accelerated catabolism of HDL in liver and/or kidney. The disorder is usually accompanied by the occurrence of premature vascular disease and a family history of coronary disease. Rare cases with severe HDL deficiency or total absence of HDL are due to mutations in genes, which encode for proteins that play a key role in HDL metabolism [apo A1, adenosine triphosphate binding cassette A1 (ABCA1), transporter APOA1/C3/A4 gene cluster, or lecithin:cholesterol acyltransferase (LCAT)].

With the application of genome-wide screening techniques, the molecular basis of some of these dyslipidaemias has been elucidated, for example, Tangier disease (Brooks-Wilson et al. 1999). Tangier disease is caused by mutations in the ABCA1 in the cell membrane. This member of a large family of transporter proteins regulates the efflux of cholesterol from peripheral cells and is the first step of 'reverse cholesterol transport (RCT)'. Tangier disease is characterized by near absence of HDL in the plasma, an accumulation of cholesteryl esters throughout the body, including tonsils and intestinal mucosa, and is usually accompanied by premature vascular disease. The next step in RCT is esterification of free cholesterol by the enzyme LCAT, present at the surface of HDL, thereby promoting the formation of mature HDL. Mutations in LCAT lead to complete or partial LCAT deficiency with the accumulation of free cholesterol and abnormal lipoproteins (the latter also known as Fish-eye disease due to the opacification of the cornea by the deposition of free cholesterol).

4.7 LPL and Apo C-II deficiency

A classic example of monogenetic lipid disorders is the chylomicro-naemia syndrome due to an inherited complete deficiency of 'clearing factor' or LPL at the vascular endothelium, leading to high plasma triglyceride levels and milky serum (Table 4.2). This condition is clinically characterized by a failure to thrive, eruptive xanthomata, lipaemia retinalis, hepatosplenomegaly, and acute pancreatitis. Inherited deficiency of the cofactor of LPL, which is necessary to activate the enzyme, apolipoprotein C-II, can cause the same clinical picture (Fojo and Brewer 1992).

4.8 Sitosterolaemia

Sitosterolaemia is a rare autosomal recessive disorder characterized by intestinal hyperabsorption of all sterols, including cholesterol and plant and shellfish sterols, and impaired ability to excrete sterols into bile. Patients with this disease have expanded body pools of cholesterol and very elevated plasma plant sterol species (sitosterol, campesterol) (>500 × normal) and frequently develop tendon and tuberous xanthomata, accelerated atherosclerosis, and premature coronary artery disease (Lu et al. 2001). This disorder is caused by mutations in other members of the ABC family, ABCG5 and ABCG8, which form a heterodimer in enterocytes and pumps sterols after absorption back into the intestinal lumen. The xanthomata in this condition resemble those in patients with homozygous FH, but their serum cholesterol levels can vary from normal to slightly elevated.

4.9 Autosomal recessive hypercholesterolaemia

Autosomal recessive hypercholesterolaemia is a rare disorder due to mutations in a protein (ARH) involved in LDL receptor-mediated endocytosis in the liver (Rader et al. 2003). This protein is one of a large family of adaptor proteins and apparently required for clustering of the LDL-receptor in the coated pit in the liver. The clearance of LDL from plasma is severely impaired. ARH is characterized by severe hypercholesterolaemia, tendon xanthomas, and premature coronary artery disease, and resembles clinically homozygous FH. The LDL-cholesterol levels tend to be intermediate between those seen in heterozygous and homozygous FH.

Table 4.2 Rare monogenetic disorders in lipid metabolism		
Disorder	**Abnormal plasma lipid**	**Cause**
Tangier disease	Low/absent HDL	Mutation in ABCA1 transporter
	Slightly increased TG	Impaired efflux cholesterol
LCAT-deficiency	Absent HDL	Mutation in LCAT
Fish-eye disease	Abnormal structure all lipoproteins	Accumulation of free cholesterol
Familial	Elevated chylomicrons/VLDL	Mutation in LPL or apoC-II
LPL- or apoC-II-deficiency	TG > 10mmol/L	Impaired clearance of chylomicrons/large VLDL particles
Sitosterolaemia	Grossly elevated plant sterols	Mutation in ABCG5 and ABCG8 transporters
	Normal to elevated TC	Increased intestinal absorption of plant sterols
		Impaired ability to excrete sterols in bile
Autosomal recessive	High LDL	Mutation in adaptor protein of
Hypercholesterolaemia (ARH)	TC > 10mmol/L	LDL-receptor
		Impaired internalization of LDL
Abetalipo-proteinaemia	Low TC (<2mmol/L) and TG (<0.5mmol/L)	Mutation in MTP
		Impaired assembly of Apo B containing lipoproteins
Hypobetalipo-proteinaemia	Low TC (< 2mmol/L) and TG (<0.5mmol/L)	Mutation in apo B100
		Impaired hepatic formation of LDL
TC: total cholesterol; TG: triglyceride		

4.10 **Abetalipoproteinaemia/ hypobetalipoproteinaemia**

Abetalipoproteinaemia is a rare autosomal recessive disease caused by mutations in the gene encoding for microsomal transfer protein, which is necessary for the assembly of chylomicrons and VLDL in the intestine and liver, respectively. Chylomicrons, VLDL, LDL, and apo B are absent from plasma. Abetalipoproteinaemia presents usually in early childhood with diarrhoea and failure to thrive and is characterized clinically by fat malabsorption, spinocerebellar degeneration, pigmented retinopathy, and acanthocytosis. Most clinical manifestations of abetalipoproteinaemia result from defects in the absorption and transport of fat-soluble vitamins for which the lipoproteins are responsible: vitamin E and to a lesser degree vitamins A and K.

Hypobetalipoproteinaemia is an autosomal dominant disorder caused by mutations in the gene that encodes for apo B100 which interfere with normal protein synthesis of apo B in the liver. The homozygous form has a clinical picture similar to abetalipoproteinaemia, but can be differentiated from abetalipoproteinaemia by family investigation: the parents of the probands with this disorder have LDL-cholesterol and apo B levels that are less than half normal, whereas parents of probands with abetalipoproteinaemia have normal lipid levels (Rader *et al.* 2003).

References

Austin MA, Hutter CM, Zimmern RL, and Humphries SE (2004). Familial hypercholesterolemia and coronary heart disease: a HuGE association review. *American Journal of Epidemiology*, **160**, 421–9.

Bourbon M, Sun XM, and Soutar AK (2007). A rare polymorphism in the low density lipoprotein (LDL) gene that affects mRNA splicing. *Atherosclerosis*, **195**, e17–e20.

Brooks-Wilson A, Marcil M, Clee SM, *et al.* (1999). Mutations in ABC1 in Tangier disease and familial high-density lipoprotein deficiency. *Nature Genetics*, **22**, 336–45.

Brunzell JD (2007). Clinical practice. Hypertriglyceridemia. *The New England Journal of Medicine*, **357**, 1009–17.

de Graaf J, Veerkamp MJ, and Stalenhoef AF (2002). Metabolic pathogenesis of familial combined hyperlipidaemia with emphasis on insulin resistance, adipose tissue metabolism and free fatty acids. *Journal of the Royal Society of Medicine*, **95**(Suppl 42), 46–53.

Fojo SS and Brewer HB (1992). Hypertriglyceridaemia due to genetic defects in lipoprotein lipase and apolipoprotein C-II. *Journal of Internal Medicine*, **231**, 669–77.

Juo SH, Bredie SJ, Kiemeney LA, Demacker PN, and Stalenhoef AF (1998). A common genetic mechanism determines plasma apolipoprotein B levels and dense LDL subfraction distribution in familial combined hyperlipidemia. *American Journal of Human Genetics*, **63**, 586–94.

Lee JC, Lusis AJ, and Pajukanta P (2006). Familial combined hyperlipidemia: upstream transcription factor 1 and beyond. *Current Opinion in Lipidology*, **17**, 101–9.

Lu K, Lee MH, Hazard S, *et al.* (2001). Two genes that map to the STSL locus cause sitosterolemia: genomic structure and spectrum of mutations involving sterolin-1 and sterolin-2, encoded by ABCG5 and ABCG8, respectively. *American Journal of Human Genetics*, **69**, 278–90.

Mahley RW and Rall SC Jr (1995). Type III hyperlipoproteinemia (Dysbetalipoproteinemia): The role of apolipoprotein E in normal and abnormal lipoprotein metabolism. In Scriver CR, *et al.*, eds. *The Metabolic Basis of Inherited Disease*, pp. 1953–73. McGraw-Hill, New York.

Rader DJ and Hobbs HH (2005). Disorders of lipoprotein metabolism. In Kasper DL, *et al.*, eds. *Harrison's Principles of Internal Medicine (on line)*, 16 edn. McGraw-Hill, New York.

Rader DJ, Cohen J, and Hobbs HH (2003). Monogenic hypercholesterolemia: new insights in pathogenesis and treatment. *Journal of Clinical Investigation*, **111**, 1795–803.

Stalenhoef AF, Demacker PN, Lutterman JA, and van't Laar A (1986). Plasma lipoproteins, apolipoproteins, and triglyceride metabolism in familial hypertriglyceridemia. *Arteriosclerosis*, **6**, 387–94.

van der Vleuten, Isaacs A, Hijmans A, van Duijn CM, Stalenhoef AF, and de Graaf J (2007). The involvement of upstream stimulatory factor 1 in Dutch patients with familial combined hyperlipidemia. *Journal of Lipid Research*, **48**, 193–200.

Veerkamp MJ, de Graaf J, Hendriks JC, Demacker PN, and Stalenhoef AF (2004). Nomogram to diagnose familial combined hyperlipidemia on the basis of results of a 5-year follow-up study. *Circulation*, **109**, 2980–5.

Chapter 5

Secondary dyslipidaemias

Rafael Carmena and José T. Real

Key points

- Secondary causes including concurrent drug therapy should be sought and excluded in patients presenting with dyslipidaemia.

- Depending on the cause, treatment is of the underlying condition, for example, hypothyroidism.

- Lipid lowering is required in addition to treatment of the underlying cause in some conditions such as diabetes, kidney disease, and HIV/AIDS.

- Dyslipidaemia is commonly seen in type 2 diabetes and metabolic syndrome, and its treatment is an important component of overall management.

5.1 Introduction

Secondary dyslipidaemias are alterations in plasma levels of lipo-proteins caused by a variety of diseases, physiological conditions (pregnancy), or external factors, such as consumption of a high fat diet. They are common and therefore become important in clinical practice. They may increase the morbidity and mortality of the pri-mary cause, as in diabetic dyslipidaemia or chronic renal failure, or complicate the evolution and treatment of a primary dyslipidaemia, such as obesity in combined familial hyperlipaemia. Not infrequently, secondary dyslipidaemias unmask the primary disease, as in the hypercholesterolaemia of hypothyroidism.

Secondary causes of dyslipidaemia should be considered before the initiation of lipid-lowering therapy. Their diagnosis is based on the coexistence of a lipid alteration and an illness or the presence of an exogenous factor capable of influencing lipid metabolism. Treat-ment should be that of the causal illness, given that dyslipidaemia is controlled or disappears when the former improves or the triggering cause is suppressed.

There are numerous causes of secondary dyslipidaemias; some of the most frequent ones are included in Table 5.1. In this chapter, we

Table 5.1 Classification of secondary hyperlipoproteinaemias by phenotype	
Phenotype	**Responsible disease or process**
I	Badly controlled diabetes mellitus
	Acute pancreatitis
	Dysgammaglobulinaemias, systemic lupus erythematosus
IIa	Hypothyroidism
	Nephrotic syndrome
	Cholestasis
	Acute intermittent porphyria
	Anorexia nervosa
	Hepatoma
	Dysgammaglobulinaemias, Werner syndrome
IIb	Nephrotic syndrome
	Oral contraception
	Dysgammaglobulinaemias
III	Hypothyroidism
	Badly controlled diabetes mellitus
	Dysgammaglobulinaemias
IV	Badly controlled diabetes mellitus
	Obesity
	Acute hepatitis
	Chronic renal deficiency
	Alcoholism
	Dysgammaglobulinaemias
	Renal transplant
	Cushing syndrome
	Burns
	Acromegaly
	Protease inhibitors (antiretroviral)

will focus only on the causes of secondary dyslipidaemias more frequently seen in clinical practice, particularly those contributing to cardiovascular risk.

5.2 **Dyslipidaemias secondary to endocrine and metabolic diseases**

5.2.1 **Diabetes mellitus (DM)**

Diabetic dyslipidaemia is defined as the association of hypertriglyceridaemia due to an increase in very low-density lipoprotein (VLDL), low high-density lipoprotein (HDL)-cholesterol (HDL-C) levels, and predominance of small and dense LDL particles in the plasma, generally with a moderate increase in LDL-cholesterol (LDL-C) and apolipoprotein B (apo B) (Carmena 1999). The prevalence of dyslipidaemia, particularly hypertriglyceridaemia with low HDL-C, is two to three times more frequent in the diabetic than in the non-diabetic population (Carmena 1999). Hypertriglyceridaemia is an independent cardiovascular risk factor in the diabetic population (Austin 1991). Furthermore, diabetes is frequently associated with increased plasma levels of LDL-C, which further contribute to the elevated cardiovascular risk observed in the diabetic population.

The prevalence of lipid alterations in type 2 DM is much more frequent (Laakso 1995) than in type 1, and are related to the presence of insulin resistance (IR) (Haffner et al. 1992). Indeed, various prospective studies have shown that fasting hyperinsulinaemia, an indirect manifestation of IR, precedes the apparition of hypertriglyceridaemia and the decrease in HDL-C (Haffner et al. 1992; Mykkanen et al. 1994). In fact, in this context of IR and metabolic syndrome, hypertriglyceridaemia may predate the onset of diabetes by many years. The elevation of plasma free fatty acids (FFA) due to IR produces two important effects on the liver: an increase in VLDL synthesis and an increase in the production of glucose (Boden 1997; Taskinen 2003). The severity of these changes is heightened by the presence of abdominal obesity, which amplifies the degree of IR (Laakso 1995; Carmena 1999). Furthermore, in the postprandial stage there is a lack of inhibition in the hepatic production of VLDL, which increases triglyceridaemia together with a prolonged postprandial lipaemia due to changes in the lipoprotein lipase (LPL), apo CIII, and apo AV (Adiels et al. 2006; Taskinen 2003). Because of these mechanisms, there are a greater number of chylomicrons and chylomicron remnants in the circulation, which are highly atherogenic (Taskinen 2003; Donnelly et al. 2005; Adiels et al. 2006).

IR is also accompanied by a greater activity of hepatic lipase and of the cholesterol ester transport protein, which explains the decrease in circulating HDL. Hypertriglyceridaemia induces frequent qualitative variations of LDL, which are enriched in triglycerides and transform into the more atherogenic small and dense LDL particles (Taskinen 2003; Adiels et al. 2006).

On the other hand, lipoproteins are glycosylated, which favours their oxidation and increases their atherogenic capacity (Taskinen 2003; Adiels et al. 2006).

The clinical consequences of diabetic dyslipidaemia are an acceleration and early appearance of arteriosclerosis and its consequences: coronary heart disease, cerebrovascular accident, and peripheral artery disease (Howard et al. 2000; Adiels et al. 2006).

With regard to diagnosis, a complete lipid profile at least once a year is recommended for all diabetics. In type 2 DM, these controls are generally conducted more often, in order to attain present recommended plasma lipid targets (American Diabetes Association 2007).

Treatment of diabetic dyslipidaemia begins with improvement and optimization of the glycaemic control, with diet therapy, regular physical aerobic exercise, and oral agents (metformin, glitazone, or sulfonylurea) or insulin if necessary (Carmena 1999; American Diabetes Association 2007). However, the majority of patients need the addition of hypolipidaemic drugs, such as statins and fibrates, in order to accomplish the therapeutic objectives (Table 5.2).

Statins have shown their efficiency in the treatment of diabetic dyslipidaemia and in lowering cardiovascular morbidity and mortality in primary and secondary prevention trials (Colhoun 2004; Cholesterol Treatment Trailist 2006) and are considered the drugs of choice.

5.2.2 **Obesity**

Central or visceral obesity is often associated with dyslipidaemia, and manifests itself as a type IV lipoprotein phenotype (hypertriglyceridaemia due to increased VLDL) and less often as IIb phenotype, with an associated elevation in cholesterol. Other alterations are a decrease in HDL-C, increase in plasma FFA, and in LDL-C (Bonora et al. 1996). Visceral obesity is defined as a waist perimeter of >102cm in males or >88cm in females, and it is related to IR (Eckel et al. 2005). The state of IR is the common denominator in a series of alterations frequently associated in clinical practice, constituting the so-called metabolic syndrome. This syndrome consists of the association of dysglycaemia, dyslipidaemia (hypertriglyceridaemia, decrease in HDL-C, and the presence of small and dense LDL), an increase of plasma FFA, hypertension, hyperuricaemia, hyperleptinaemia, and elevated PA-1, amongst others (Eckel et al. 2005).

The increased flow of FFA to the liver, characteristic of visceral obesity, has been shown to increase apo B synthesis, which in turn increases the number of VLDL particles secreted by the liver, causing hypertriglyceridaemia (Ascaso et al. 1997; Nielson and Jenson 1997). As was the case in type 2 DM, the decrease in HDL-C is due to the combination of decreased LPL activity (associated with lower HDL synthesis), and an increase in LH activity, which accelerates hepatic HDL catabolism (Taskinen 2003; Adiels et al. 2006).

60

Table 5.2 **Lipid objectives for primary and secondary prevention in diabetes mellitus**		
	No CHD	**CHD**
CT	<200	<200
cLDL	<100	<70
TG	<200	<150
cHDL	>40	>40
Figures in mg/dL. CHD = coronary heart disease.		

The initial therapeutic step for dyslipidaemia in obesity consists of weight loss through a low calorie diet and physical aerobic exercise (Carmena *et al.* 1984). It may be necessary to add statins or fibrates, according to the lipoprotein phenotype presented. The new endocannabinoid receptor blocker rimonabant has also been shown to improve the lipid profile in obese subjects (Christensen *et al.* 2007).

5.2.3 **Hypothyroidism**

Hypercholesterolaemia due to elevated LDL-C is not an infrequent early manifestation in adult hypothyroidism, particularly in menopausal women with autoimmune thyroiditis. A high level of suspicion (measurement of TSH) is therefore required in the lipid clinic. If untreated, elevated LDL-C will further contribute to the high coronary risk observed in these patients.

The prevalence of dyslipidaemia in primary hypothyroidism is elevated, being present is as many as 80–85% of patients with clinical hypothyroidism (Abrams and Grundy 1981). It has been found that up to 20% of women older than 40yrs and with severe type IIa dyslipidaemia (total cholesterol >300mg/dL) have hypothyroidism (Abrams and Grundy 1981). The most constant lipid alteration is hypercholesterolaemia due to an increase in LDL-C, which is detected in almost 80% of cases. Hypertriglyceridaemia is detected in less than half of the cases, commonly associated with hypercholesterolaemia (Abrams and Grundy 1981).

The dyslipidaemia secondary to hypothyroidism is explained by a reduction in the clearance of LDL particles through the LDL receptor pathway, due to a decrease in its number and function. These abnormalities are reverted once replacement therapy with levothyroxine is initiated (Hylander and Rosenqvist 1982). A decrease in LPL activity in plasma, adipose tissue, and liver has also been advocated and would explain hypertriglyceridaemia in some cases. Failure to diagnose hypothyroidism and initiation of statin therapy for hypercholesterolaemia is a frequent cause of myalgia and myopathy.

5.2.4 **Cushing's syndrome and treatment with glucocorticoids**

Hypercortisolism, produced by the endogenous overproduction of glucocorticoids (Cushing's syndrome) or, more frequently, by the exogenous administration of glucocorticoids, is frequently associated with increased LDL-C. Common features of hypercortisolism states are visceral obesity with IR, dysglycaemia, and increased hepatic VLDL production. Thus, there is often an associated increase in triglycerides, particularly when diabetes is induced by the glucocorticoid excess (Pedersen *et al.* 1994).

5.3 **Dyslipidaemias secondary to drugs and toxins**

5.3.1 **High alcohol consumption**

Alcohol consumption and abuse is, together with diabetes and obesity, one of the most frequent causes of secondary dyslipidaemias (Lieber 1985). Its predominant effect is to produce hypertriglyceridaemia. Alcohol alters the lipid metabolism through two different mechanisms: direct action on the hepatic parenchyma and triggering of metabolic changes, which appear as a consequence of the catabolism of ethanol (Schapiro *et al.* 1965). The hepatic oxidation of ethanol is carried out as a priority, and has preference over that of other substrates, such as FFA, lactate, or glucose. Approximately 80% of oxidized ethanol in the liver is released into the systemic circulation in the form of acetate, which inhibits the oxidation of the lipids in peripheral tissues (Schapiro *et al.* 1965). Ethanol increases the rate of lipolysis and enhances the flux of FFA to the liver, resulting in increased VLDL and triglyceride synthesis (Schapiro *et al.* 1965), and a type IV phenotype. If the clearance of triglyceride-rich particles is delayed, then a type V phenotype will supervene due to the accumulation of chylomicrons. On the other hand, if the hepatic production of apo B100 does not increase sufficiently, then the excess fat will generate hepatic steatosis (Chait *et al.* 1972).

The treatment of alcoholic hypertriglyceridaemia is based on the suppression of ethanol consumption. In some cases, the use of fibrates, ω-3 fatty acids, or nicotinic acid, may be indicated.

Moderate regular alcohol intake produces a slight increase in serum HDL and apo AI and AII concentrations, possibly by inducing hepatic microsomal enzymes, and could have a cardioprotective effect (Fan 2007). On the other hand, excessive alcohol consumption is an important risk factor for hypertension, liver disease, and low-serum HDL levels.

5.3.2 **Oral contraception**

The use of oral contraceptives is associated with dyslipidaemia and an increased risk of cardiovascular diseases, due to the adverse plasma lipid and glucose changes and the tendency to raise blood pressure (Durrington 2007).

The most common lipid disorder in women using hormonal contraception is hypertriglyceridaemia (phenotype IV), which is related to the oestrogen content in the preparation, the quantity of progestogens, and the plasma triglyceride levels before treatment. Oestrogen increases the hepatic synthesis of triglycerides and VLDL, and can produce IR. Progestogens raise serum cholesterol at the expense of LDL-C (Godsland *et al.* 1990, Kwok *et al.* 2004). Therefore, in clinical practice, the prescription of female sexual hormones requires the control of plasma lipids to detect undesired effects. According to the preparations used and depending on the concentration of oestrogen or progestogen, different phenotypes can appear (Godsland et al. 1990, Walsh 1993).

Orally administered oestrogens and, to a lesser degree, those administered by transdermic route in menopausal women, reduce LDL-C by increasing the LDL receptor activity and increase HDL-C plasma concentration (Godsland et al. 1990). These changes, however, are not accompanied by a reduction in cardiovascular morbidity and mortality in menopausal women and should not be used to this end.

5.3.3 **Antiretroviral treatment**

Patients infected by the human immunodeficiency virus (HIV 1) show changes in the lipid profile, which are characterized by hypertriglyce-ridaemia and a reduction in HDL-C. These changes are due to effects of the viral infection itself, the acute phase reactants, and the action of the circulating cytokines (Carr et al. 1999).

Highly active antiretroviral therapy has been shown to induce IR, secondary dyslipidaemia and changes in the distribution of body fat (lipodystrophy), increasing fat deposits in breasts, back (buffalo hump) and abdomen, and reducing subcutaneous fat deposits in the face and other body areas (Carr et al. 1999). In these patients, severe hypertriglyceridaemia and low HDL-C are observed, and are related to the use of protease inhibitors (mainly ritonavir), which act by selectively blocking the proteosome degradation of the apo B (Pur-nell et al. 2000, Lenhard et al. 2000). Since control of HIV infection is mandatory antiretroviral therapy cannot be discontinued although ritonavir can be substituted with efavirenz, which has been shown to induce less lipid changes (Carr et al. 1999).

In these patients, lifestyle changes and diet therapy have little or no effect on lipodystrophy and dyslipidaemia. Treatment with fibrates associated with ω-3 fatty acids has been shown to be useful. In gener-al, the use of statins increases the risk of secondary muscular effects, as the protease inhibitors also use the cytochrome P4503A4. Fluvasta-tin and pravastatin, which are metabolized by different systems, are the prefered statins that can be prescribed in these patients.

5.3.4 **Other drugs**

Table 5.3 includes a summary of some of the drugs most frequently involved in dyslipidaemia (Lithell 1993).

5.4 **Renal diseases**

5.4.1 **Nephrotic syndrome**

Hypercholesterolaemia frequently exists in nephrotic syndrome due to an increase in levels of LDL-C (IIa phenotype), associated with the

Table 5.3 Lipid changes induced by drugs		
Drug	**Lipoprotein alterations**	**Phenotype**
Beta blockers (sympathico-mimetic intrinsic activity)	↑ VLDL, ↓ HDL, LDL N ↑ o N VLDL, HDL N, LDL N	IV
Thiazides	↑ VLDL, ↑ LDL, HDL N	IIB
Oestrogen	↑ VLDL, o N LDL, ↑ HDL	IIB
Progesterone	↑ VLDL ↑LDL, ↓ HDL	IIB, IV
Androgens	↑ LDL, ↓ HDL, ↓ VLDL	IIA
Corticoids	VLDL, ↑ LDL, HDL	IIB, IV
Retinoic acid	↑VLDL, LDL N, HDL N	IV
Amiodarone	↑ LDL, HDL N, VLDL N	IIA
Ciclosporin	↑ LDL, VLDL N, HDL N	IIA
Protease inhibitors (antiretroviral)	↑↑ VLDL, LDL N, ↓ HDL	IV
Hepatic microsomal inductors (phenobarbital, rifampicin, phenytoin, etc.)	↑VLDL, ↑ LDL, ↑↑HDL	IIB

well-known reduction of plasma albumin. Occasionally, hypertriglyc-eridaemia (IIb phenotype), can also be seen. Plasma Lp(a) levels raise significantly in relation to the degree of proteinuria (Joven et al. 1990).

The mechanisms responsible for dyslipidaemia include an increase in VLDL hepatic synthesis, probably related to the increase of the FFA not bound to the albumin, a decrease in LDL catabolism mediated by the LDL receptor, and an increase in the hepatic pro-duction of apo B. There is also a direct hepatic secretion of LDL related to the reduced levels of albumin (Joven et al. 1990, Grundy 1989). Hypertriglyceridaemia is explained by the decrease in LPL activity and the increase in VLDL secretion.

Statins, which are eliminated almost exclusively through the bile duct, are the treatment of choice (Grundy 1989). Combination with ω-3 fatty acids could be a good option in cases of phenotype IIb that do not respond to monotherapy with statins. Fibrates could only be used, if at all, at half dosage and with extreme caution, due to the well-known risk of myopathy in these patients (Grundy 1989).

5.4.2 **Chronic kidney disease**

The dyslipidaemia of chronic kidney disease is characterized by hypertriglyceridaemia with an increase in the VLDL and LDL triglyce-ride content, a decrease in HDL-C and a predominance of small and dense LDL particles. The pathophysiological mechanisms are complex and include lowering of LPL activity combined with an increase in CEPT and LH activities (Bergesio et al. 1992).

Haemodialysis, with the administration of heparin, further depletes LPL and LH, and contributes to the worsening of hypertriglyceridaemia (Bergesio *et al.* 1992). In these patients, the origin of dyslipidaemia is very complex, as it often coexists with other causes of alterations in lipid metabolism such as weight gain, corticosteroid treatment, antihypertensive agents, etc.

In addition to dietary changes, statins are the drugs of choice to treat these patients. The administration of statins has shown to significantly reduce the deterioration of renal function and the cardiovascular risk (Shepherd *et al.* 2007). Dyslipidaemia is also improved by renal transplantation.

5.5 **Liver disorders**

5.5.1 **Cholestasis**

Primary or secondary cholestasis can produce extreme hypercholesterolaemia due to the formation of a special particle, known as lipoprotein X (LpX), which contains 25% of free cholesterol, 60% phospholipids, and is virtually devoid of triglycerides (Sabesin 1980). The origin of LpX is still unknown; the reflux of biliary cholesterol and/or phospholipids, and some degree of LCAT deficiency could be involved (Sabesin 1980).

A common example of this type of dyslipidaemia is that seen in primary biliary cirrhosis, classically accompanied by xanthomas and xanthelasmas. In this condition, however, hypercholesterolaemia is not associated with premature atherosclerosis and it has been advocated that LpX reduces the atherogenicity of LDL-C by preventing LDL oxidation (Su 2007).

LpX disappears with the relief of biliary obstruction. When this is not possible, as in primary biliary cirrhosis, treatment includes diet and administration of colestyramine or ursodeoxycholic acid. Statins should be avoided, due to the increased risk of myopathy. LDL apheresis may be necessary in severe and resistant cases (Durrington 2007).

References

Abrams JJ and Grundy SM (1901). Cholesterol metabolism in hypothyroidism and hyperthyrodism in man. *Journal of Lipid Research*, **22**, 323–38.

Adiels M, Olofsson SO, Taskinen MR, and Boren J (2006). Diabetic dyslipemia. *Current Opinion in Lipidology*, **17**, 238–46.

American Diabetes Association (2007). Standards of medical care in diabetes. *Diabetes Care*, **30**, S4–S41.

Ascaso JF, Sales J, Merchante A, et al. (1997). Influence of obesity on plasma lipoproteins, glycaemia and insulinaemia in patients with familial combined hyperlipidaemia. *International Journal of Obesity-Related Metabolic Disorders*, **21**, 360–66.

Austin MA. (1991). Plasma triglyceride and coronary heart disease. *Arteriosclerosis Thrombosis*, **11**, 2–14.

Bergesio F, Monzani G, Ciuti R et al. (1992). Lipids and apolipoproteins change during the progression of chronic renal failure. *Clin Nephrol* **38**: 264–270.

Boden G. (1997). Role of fatty acids in the pathogenesis of insulin resistance and NIDDM. *Diabetes,* **46**, 3–10.

Bonora E, Targher G, Branzi P, et al. (1996). Cardiovascular risk profile in 38-years and in 18-years old men. Contribution of body fat content and regional fat distribution. *International Journal of Obesity-Related Metabolic Disorders*, **20**, 28–36.

Carmena R (1999). Dislipemia diabética. In Ediciones Doyma SA, Barcelona, R Carmena and y JM Ordovas, eds. Hiperlipemias. Clínica y Tratamiento. pp. 139–153.

Carmena R, Ascaso JF, Tebar J, and Soriano J. (1984). Changes in plasma high-density lipoproteins after body weight reduction in obese women. *International Journal of Obesity* **8**, 135-40.

Carr A, Samaras K, Thorisdottir A et al. (1999). Diagnosis,prediction and natural course of HIV-1 protease inhibition associated lipodystrophy, hyperlipemia and diabetes mellitus: a cohort study. *Lancet* **353**, 2093–9.

Chait A, Mancini M, February AW, Lewis B (1972). Clinical and metabolic study of alcoholic hyperlipidemia. *Lancet* **2**, 62-64.

Cholesterol Treatment Trialist (CTT) Collaborators (2008). Efficacy of cholesterol-lowering therapy in 18,686 people with diabetes in 14 randomised trials of statins: a meta-analysis. *Lancet*, **371**, 117–25.

Christensen R, Kristensen PK, Bartels EM, Bliddal H, and Astrup A (2007). Efficacy and safety of the weight-loss drug rimonabant: a meta-analysis of randomised trials. *The Lancet,* **370**, 1706–13.

Colhoun HM, Betteridge DJ, Durrington PN, et al. (2004). Primary prevention of cardiovascular disease with atorvastatin in type 2 diabetes in the collaborative atorvastatin diabetes study (CARDS). A multicentre randomized placebo-controlled trial. *Lancet,* **364**, 685–96.

Donnelly KL, Smith CI, Schwarzenberg SJ, et al. (2005). Sources of fatty acids stored in liver and secreted via lipoproteins in patients with nonalcoholic fatty liver disease. *Journal of Clinical Investigations* **115**, 1343–51.

Durrington PN (2007). Secondary hyperlipidaemia. In: *Hyperlipidemia. Diagnosis and management 3rd* edition. PN Durrington, Hodder Arnold, London; 310–359.

Eckel RH, Grundy SM, and Zimmet PZ (2005). The metabolic syndrome. *The Lancet,* **365**, 1415–28.

Fan AZ (2007). Association of lifetime alcohol drinking trajectories with cardiometabolic risk. *J Clin Endocrinol Metab* **20**.

Godsland IF, Crook D, Simpson R et al. (1990). The effects of different formulations of oral contraceptive agents on lipid and carbohydrate metabolism. *N Engl J Med* **323**, 1375–81.

Grundy SM, Vega GL (1989). Rationale and management of hyperlipidemia of the nephrotic syndrome. *Am J Med* **7**, 3N–11N

Haffner SM, Valdez RA, Hazuda HP, Mitchell BD, Morales PA, and Stern MP (1992). Prospective analysis of the insulin-resistance syndrome (Syndrome X). *Diabetes*, **41**, 715–22.

Howard BV, Robbins DC, Sievers ML, et al. (2000). LDL cholesterol as a strong predictor of coronary heart disease in diabetic individuals with insulin resistance and low LDL: the Strong Heart Study. *Arteriosclerosis Thrombosis Vascular Biology*, **20**, 830–5.

Hylander B, Rosenqvist U (1982). Time course effect of thyroxine on serum lipoprotein concentrations in hypothyroid subjects. *Acta Med Scand*, **211**, 287–91.

Joven J, Villabona C, Vilella E, Masana L, Albertí R, Vallés M (1990). Abnormalities of lipoprotein metabolism in patients with the nephrotic syndrome. *N Engl J Med* **323**, 579–584.

Kwok S, Selby PL, McElduff P et al. (2004). Progestogens of varying androgenicity and cardiovascular risk factors in postmenopausal women receiving oestrogen replacement therapy. *Clin Endocrinol* **61**, 760–7.

Laakso M (1995). Epidemiology of diabetic dyslipidemia. *Diabetes Review*, **3**, 408–22.

Lenhard JM, Croom DK, Weiel JE, Winegar DA (2000). HIV protease inhibitors stimulate hepatic triglyceride synthesis. *Arterioscler Thromb Vasc Biol* **20**, 2625–9.

Lieber CS (1985). Alcohol and the liver: metabolism of ethanol, metabolic effects and pathogenesis of injury. *Acta Med Scand* **703**, 11–55.

Lithell H (1993). Hypertension and hyperlipemia. A review. *Am J Hypertens* **6**, 303S–308S.

Mykkanen L, Kuusito J, Haffner SM, Pyörälä K, and Lakkso M (1994). Hyperinsulinemia predicts multiple atherogenic changes in lipoproteins in elderly subjects. *Arteriosclerosis Thrombosis*, **14**, 518–26.

Nielsen S and Jensen MD (1997). Obesity and cardiovascular disease: is body structure a factor?. *Current Opinion in Lipidology* **4**, 200–204.

Pedersen SB, Jonler M, Richelsen B (1994). Characterization of regional and gender differences in glucocorticoid receptors and lipoprotein lipase activity in human adipose tissue. *J Clin Endocrinol Metab* **78**, 1354–1359.

Purnell JQ, Zambon A, Knopp RH et al. (2000). Effect of ritonavir on lipids and postheparin lipase activity in normal subjects. *AIDS* **14**, 51–7.

Sabesin SM, Bertram PD, Freeman MR (1980). Lipoprotein metabolism in liver disease. *Adv Intern Med* **25**, 117–46.

Schapiro RH, Scheig RL, Drurumey GD, Mendelson JH, Isselbacher KJ (1965). Effect of prolonged ethanol ingestion on the transport and metabolism of lipids in man. *N Engl J Med* **272**, 610–615.

Shepherd J, Kastelein JJ, Bittner V *et al.*; Treating to New Targets Investigators (2007). Effect of intensive lipid lowering with atorvastatin on renal function in patients with coronary heart disease: the Treating to New Targets (TNT) study. *Clin J Am Soc Nephrol* **2**, 1131–9.

Su TC, Hwang JJ, Kao JH (2007). Hypercholesterolemia in primary biliary cirrhosis. *N Eng J Med* **357**, 1561–62.

Taskinen MR (2003). Diabetic dyslipidemia: from basic research to clinical practice. *Diabetologia*, **46**, 733–49.

Walsh BW, Sack FM (1993). Effects of low dose oral contraceptives on VLDL and LDL metabolism. *J Clin Invest* **91**, 2126–2132.

Chapter 6

Diet and lifestyle

Jonathan Morrell and Jacqueline Morrell

Key points

- Consume a healthy, balanced diet.
- Aim for a healthy body weight and shape.
- Reduce saturated and trans fats and substitute with non-hydrogenated, unsaturated fats. Choose whole grains as the main form of carbohydrates, and consume a diet high in fruit and vegetables.
- Be physically active.
- Avoid use of (and exposure to) tobacco products.

6.1 Introduction

Despite the major advances of clinical medicine, maintaining a healthy diet and lifestyle offers the greatest potential for reducing the risk of cardiovascular disease (CVD) in populations. Even for individuals, appropriate diet and lifestyle remain the foundation of clinical intervention for prevention.

Multiple diet and lifestyle factors influence the development of CVD and its risk factors and yet the vast majority of research studies have focused on individual dietary and lifestyle components and few studies examine the effect of a comprehensive approach. This chapter aims to review the components of a healthy diet and lifestyle, which contribute to cardiovascular health and identify some of the practical steps required for their implementation.

6.2 The components of a healthy lifestyle

6.2.1 Balance calorie intake and physical activity to maintain a healthy body weight and shape

To avoid weight gain, individuals must balance energy intake with energy expenditure.

Over the past 20yrs, the number of overweight and obese people has reached epidemic proportions in many countries. Both increased total adiposity [measured by body mass index (BMI)] and visceral adiposity (measured by waist hip ratio or waist circumference) increase the risk of CVD. Centrally obese individuals often show features of the metabolic syndrome including, small dense low-density lipoprotein (LDL) cholesterol, low high-density lipoprotein (HDL) cholesterol, raised triglycerides, elevated blood pressure and impaired glucose regulation. Weight reduction is appropriate for those who are overweight (BMI $\geq25kg/m^2$) or for those with increased waist circumference (≥102cm in men, ≥88cm in women). Energy dense foods such as saturated fats and refined carbohydrates are targets for reduction but a balanced, healthy eating plan that is mildly hypocaloric, allows moderate fat and a variety of food choices has more chance of compliance than a typical low-fat diet. All adults should accumulate ≥30min of physical activity on most days of the week but more activity is associated with increased benefits and ≥60min is required when losing weight. Overweight people should aim to lose around 0.5kg per week. These changes are not easy and require sustained personal and family motivation and appropriate professional support.

6.2.2 **Limit intake of saturated and trans fats and cholesterol**

Geographic and migration studies have confirmed the link between intake of saturated fat, cholesterol levels, and CVD mortality. Prospective studies, such as the Nurses' Health Study show that higher intakes of both saturated and trans fats are associated with increased risk, whereas higher intakes of the unsaturated fats (polyunsaturates and monounsaturates) are associated with decreased risk. Mensink's meta-analysis of 27 feeding studies shows the relative effects on lipoproteins of different fatty acids, when substituted isocalorically for carbohydrates (Figure 6.1).

As a result of these studies, guidelines recommend limiting saturated fat intake to <7–10% and trans fats to <1% of the 25–35% dietary energy content which fat should contribute to a healthy diet. Health professionals and patients, however, find these numerical criteria difficult to interpret and recommendations to reduce saturated and trans fats should be practically based. Reducing saturated fats largely involves choosing lean meat and low-fat dairy products and reducing trans fats essentially means avoiding commercially fried and baked products. Responsible manufacturers are now producing virtually trans fat-free products but some trans fats are unavoidable as they occur naturally in dairy products.

The second major strategy to limit the intake of saturated and trans fats involves substituting them with unsaturated fats. A meta-analysis of trials of reducing saturated fat by using monounsaturated or polyunsaturated fats as a replacement has shown a risk reduction for CVD events of 24%.

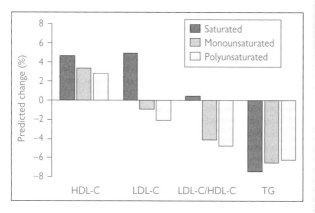

Figure 6.1 Predicted changes in serum lipids and lipoproteins with specific fatty acids, substituted under iso-caloric conditions. (*Mensink Arterioscler Thromb* 1992; **12**: 911–919). Figure from: Hu F and Willett W. Optimal Diets for Prevention of Coronary Heart Disease. *JAMA* 2002; **288**: 2569–2578

Several prospective studies have shown an inverse association between nut consumption and CVD. Although high in fat, the predominant fats in nuts such as almonds and walnuts are unsaturated and therefore lower LDL cholesterol.

Dietary cholesterol also raises total and LDL cholesterol levels. There is a wide interindividual variation in the amount absorbed but as the amounts are usually small this means reducing saturated fat is a far more potent intervention to reduce serum cholesterol.

6.2.3 Consume fish, especially oily fish at least twice a week

The two major types of polyunsaturated fatty acids, delineated by the position of the double bond nearest to the methyl end of the fatty acid chain, are omega-3 fatty acids and omega-6 fatty acids. Linoleic acid (found in vegetable oils such as sunflower, soya bean, and corn) is the principal omega-6 fatty acid and, similar to all fatty acids, is a structural lipid and a source of energy. In addition, it is an essential fatty acid involved in the manufacture of prostaglandins and leukotrienes. Most people achieve adequate amounts. Intake of linoleic acid is usually recommended not to exceed 10% of dietary energy largely due to the lack of long-term safety assurance despite evidence for improved lipids with higher amounts.

Alpha-linolenic acid (ALA—found in rapeseed [canola], flaxseed, soya bean oils and algae) is the plant precursor of the omega-3 group and the Lyon Diet Heart Study showed reductions in coronary and all-cause mortality in CHD patients who ate a diet enriched with ALA. Fish feeding on ALA-containing plankton produce other omega-3 fatty acids, chiefly eicosapentaenoic acid (EPA) and docosahexaenoic acid (DHA). EPA and DHA are technically not essential fatty acids as small amounts can be formed in the body from ALA. The amounts formed, however, are probably insufficient for a cardioprotective effect in most people. Both epidemiological studies of fish consumers and randomized clinical trials of fish or supplement consumption have shown reductions in coronary and total mortality, and particularly, sudden death. The mechanisms are unknown but omega-3 fatty acids may have anti-arrhythmic, anti-thrombotic, anti-inflammatory, and anti-atherosclerotic actions. High dose omega-3 fatty acids will reduce triglyceride levels. Eating fish (particularly oily fish, rich in EPA and DHA) is another way of displacing saturated fats from the diet and guidelines recommend two servings of fish ($2 \times 100g$) a week.

The optimal balance between omega-6 and omega-3 fatty acids remains unresolved and some have proposed increasing the amount of omega-3 fatty acids at the expense of linoleic acid. As both have separate mechanisms for reducing CVD risk, it seems sensible to increase omega-3 intake without decreasing linoleic acid.

6.2.4 **Consume a diet rich in fruits and vegetables**

Observational studies have shown lower risk of CVD in people who consume a diet rich in fruits and vegetables, and short-term trials have shown improvement in CVD risk factors, such as blood pressure. Fruits and vegetables are low in energy density and are therefore very useful in weight-reducing diets. They are often high in fibre and contain multiple micronutrients. The mechanisms of benefit are obscure but include either positive benefits of macro- or micronutrients or just the displacement of other foods from the diet.

Although epidemiologic evidence suggests that a high intake of antioxidant vitamins (such as vitamin E, C, and β-carotene) is associated with lower CVD risk, trials of antioxidant supplements show no benefit and supplements are not recommended. CVD risk reduction with folic acid supplementation has also been disappointing. Naturally occurring polyphenols, especially flavonoids, found in grapes, olive oil, and tea, may be more effective but definitive recommendations are awaited. For the time being, a variety of fruits and vegetables are recommended, particularly those that are highly coloured (green leafy vegetables, berries, fruits) whose micronutrient content is higher. In addition, preparation techniques should preserve the micronutrient and fibre content without adding unnecessary calories, fats, sugar, or salt.

6.2.5 **Choose whole-grain, high-fibre foods**

The consumption of a diet high in the complex carbohydrates found in whole-grain products and fibre is associated with reduced CVD. Part of the effect comes from insoluble fibre, which promotes satiety by slowing gastric emptying and helps to control energy intake and therefore, weight. Soluble or viscous fibre, such as β-glucan or pectin, modestly reduces LDL cholesterol by about 2–3%.

Most cereal grains are highly processed before consumption, increasing their starch content but reducing their content of fibre, essential fatty acids, and other micronutrients. Starchy foods made from refined grains, such as white bread, are rapidly digested to glucose inducing rapid glycaemic and insulinaemic responses and are said to have a high glycaemic index (GI). Unrefined, whole-grain products (e.g., whole wheat, oats, barley, brown rice, and bulgar wheat) have a slower rate of digestion and lower GI values, which may also contribute to benefit.

6.2.6 **Choose and prepare foods with little or no salt**

There is a progressive dose–response relationship between sodium intake and blood pressure. Reduced intake reduces the risk of CVD, can prevent hypertension (particularly in older people), and lower blood pressure in treated patients. Diets rich in potassium (found in fruits and vegetables) offset the effect of high sodium.

Three-quarters of the salt we eat is already in the food we buy, so reducing sodium intake means making appropriate choices both in shops and food outlets as well as in the kitchen and on the table.

6.2.7 **Consume alcohol in moderation**

Many studies show that moderate alcohol drinking is associated with a reduced risk of CVD. The studies are difficult to interpret because of the influence of people who have stopped drinking for health reasons. Also, because of the many hazards of high alcohol consumption, drinking alcohol is not recommended for health reasons. High alcohol consumption is a common reason for hypertriglyceridaemia. If alcohol is to be consumed, levels associated with the epidemiology would suggest no more than two drinks a day.

6.2.8 **Avoid use of and exposure to tobacco products**

There is overwhelming evidence for the adverse effects of tobacco and secondary exposure to tobacco smoke. The effects relate to the amount and duration of exposure. All smokers should be professionally encouraged to permanently stop smoking (Ask, Assess, Advise, Assist, and Arrange).

6.3 **Other dietary factors**

6.3.1 **Soy protein**

In people with high cholesterol, a large amount of soy protein (25g/day) may lower LDL cholesterol by up to 6%. How much of this relates to substitution of animal fats and how much to a direct effect is unclear.

6.3.2 **Plant sterols**

Plant sterols are analogues of cholesterol, providing structural integrity to cell membranes as well as being a starting material for hormones. Small amounts exist naturally in the diet but larger amounts (around 2g/day) can lower LDL cholesterol by 10%. Both unsaturated plant sterols and saturated plant stanols are incorporated into a variety of foods such as spreads, yoghurts, mini-drinks, milk, and orange juice and their effects are almost identical. When recommended, the energy content of each food should be taken into account and long-term compliance is required. At present, plant sterols have no CVD outcome data.

A number of studies have combined the cholesterol-lowering properties of a number of foods in a 'portfolio' approach. A low fat diet enriched with plant sterols, soy protein, soluble fibre, and almonds lowered LDL cholesterol by 29%, equivalent to a low dose statin.

6.4 **Putting it all together**

Diet and lifestyle modifications can effectively alter CVD risk factors and lower CVD risk. Combining dietary and lifestyle changes is more effective than modifying any single factor alone. Analyses from the Nurses' Health Study showed that 74% of CHD events could be prevented by not smoking, eating a healthy diet, maintaining a healthy body weight, exercising regularly, and being prudent with alcohol. Changes in sodium and saturated fat intake, smoking, and vegetable consumption in North Karelia, Finland, have more than halved CVD. Change to low-fat vegetarian diet, moderate aerobic exercise, smoking cessation, and psychological support could reduce LDL cholesterol by 37.2% and angiographically reduce the progression of disease. A caveat here is that low-fat regimens are hard to follow and have been replaced by changes in the types of fats consumed as described earlier. The Lyon Diet Heart Study impressively reduced CHD death by more than 70% using a Mediterranean diet enriched by alpha linolenic acid.

Changing diet and lifestyle patterns would fail if information was not clearly understood and expressed in a meaningful way to patients. Approaches such as the 'Eatwell' plate have proved successful in demonstrating the relative proportions of the major dietary components. A number of practical tips to implement diet and lifestyle recommendations are shown in Table 6.1.

Table 6.1 Practical tips

Lifestyle

- Know your energy needs to achieve and maintain a healthy weight
- Work out the energy content of the food and drinks you consume
- Monitor your energy intake, weight, and physical activity (pedometer)
- Monitor inactivity (TV, computer)
- Incorporate physical activity into everyday activities
- Avoid tobacco
- Drink alcohol in moderation

Food choices and preparation

- Food choices and preparation
- Prepare and eat smaller portions, use smaller plates

How do I know if saturated fat is high?

High	Low
>5g/100g	1.5g/100g

How do I know if salt is high?

High	Low
>1.5g/100g (or 0.6g sodium)	≤0.3g/100g (or 0.1g sodium)

- Eat a variety of fresh, frozen, or canned foods
- Avoid processed foods that are often high in fats, salt, and sugars
- Cut back on pastries and high-calorie bakery products
- Replace high-calorie snack foods with fruit and vegetables
- Limit food and drinks high in added sugars
- Increase fibre intake by eating legumes, whole grain products, fruit, and vegetables
- Use lean cuts of meat and remove skin from poultry
- Grill, bake or griddle fish, meat or poultry, steam vegetables
- Incorporate vegetable-based meat substitutes into favourite recipes
- Use liquid vegetable oils rather than solid fats
- Use dairy products that are low-fat or fat-free
- Reduce salt intake by choosing low- or no-salt products, limiting condiments and avoiding in cooking

6.5 **Summary**

A variety of options now exist for designing attractive and CVD-friendly diets. The diet should include healthy types of fat and carbohydrate and balance energy intake and expenditure. Together with regular physical activity, avoidance of tobacco and maintaining a healthy weight, such interventions may prevent the majority of CVD in western populations.

References

JBS2 (2005). Joint British Societies' guidelines on prevention of cardiovascular disease in clinical practice. *Heart*, **91**(Suppl V), v1–v52.

Fourth Joint Task Force of the European Society of Cardiology and Other Societies on Cardiovascular Disease Prevention in Clinical Practice (2007). European guidelines on cardiovascular disease prevention in clinical practice: executive summary. *European Heart Journal*, **28**, 2375–414.

Lichtenstein AH, Appel LJ, Brands M *et al.* (2006). Diet and Lifestyle Recommendations Revision (2006). A Scientific Statement from the American Heart Association Nutrition Committee. *Circulation*, **114**, 82–96.

Diets consistent with the recommendations exemplified in this chapter are DASH (Dietary Approaches to Stop Hypertension) http://www.nhlbi.nih.gov/health/public/heart/hbp/dash and TLC (Therapeutic Lifestyle Changes) http://www.nhlbi.nih.gov/cgi-bin/chd/step2intro.cgi

Mensink RB, Katan MB (1992). Effect of dietary fatty accids on serum lipids and lipoproteins. A meta-analysis of 27 trials. *Arteriosclerosis and Thrombosis*, **12**, 911–9.

Chapter 7

Pharmacological therapy: statins

D. John Betteridge

> ### Key points
>
> - Statins are potent, competitive inhibitors of the rate-determining step in cholesterol synthesis which leads to up-regulation of hepatic LDL-receptor activity and decrease in plasma LDL.
> - There is a huge database of information from RCTS in both primary and secondary CVD prevention and in a wide range of patient groups on which to base therapy.
> - Statins are the most potent agents for reducing LDL and are first-line therapy for the great majority of patients.
> - Statins are safe and well tolerated, and myositis and abnormal liver function are exceedingly rare.

7.1 Introduction

Pharmacological treatment of dyslipidaemia has progressed enormously in the past two decades such that it has become one of the most successful of all therapeutic strategies. Data available from randomized, controlled, clinical trials (RCTS) allow the clinician to make informed, evidence-based, treatment decisions in many groups of patients. Importantly, benefits go beyond the surrogates of changes in plasma lipid and lipoprotein concentrations to the real target, the reduction of the clinical consequences of atherosclerotic vascular disease. These landmark developments are largely due to the introduction of the statins in 1985. These drugs proved to be highly effective in lowering plasma low density lipoprotein (LDL) and, in addition, safe and well tolerated. The availability of the statins enabled, for the first time, definitive trials to be undertaken to test the potential of LDL-lowering for the reduction of vascular events and mortality.

The importance of the enzyme, 3-hydoxy-3-methylglutaryl coenzyme A (HMG-CoA) reductase in cholesterol homoeostasis was becoming established in the 1960s and 1970s and prompted a search for inhibitors of the enzyme. It was the pioneering work of Akira Endo which produced the prototype statin, compactin (not developed for general use), isolated from the culture broth of penicillium citrinum (Endo 1992).

7.2 **Mechanism of action**

Statins are specific, competitive inhibitors of HMG-CoA reductase which catalyses the first committed step in cholesterol synthesis, the conversion of HMG-CoA to mevalonate. They are extremely potent, with inhibitory constants of around 10^9 molar. Inhibition (approximately 40% *in vivo*) of cholesterol synthesis induces a series of reactions to restore cellular cholesterol homeostasis involving a family of regulatory proteins, sterol regulatory element binding proteins (SREBPs). SREBPs control the transcription of key enzymes and proteins in cholesterol metabolism including the LDL-receptor. Reduced intracellular cholesterol promotes cleavage of the membrane-bound SREBP, which releases the active transcription factor which translocates to the nucleus, enhancing the transcription of the LDL-receptor (Brown and Goldstein 1997). The liver is the major organ for cholesterol synthesis and for LDL catabolism, and hepatic LDL activity is a major determinant of plasma LDL and apoprotein B concentrations. Kinetic studies *in vivo* have demonstrated that statins stimulate LDL catabolism and other lipoproteins of the VLDL cascade such as remnant particles (Gaw *et al.* 1993; Vega *et al.* 1998).

7.3 **Pharmacology**

The first statins, lovastatin, simvastatin, and pravastatin, were derived from fungal metabolites. Subsequently, synthetic statins, fluvastatin, atorvastatin, rosuvastatin, and pitavastatin (available in Japan) have been introduced. They have in common a dihydroxy heptenoic side chain responsible for binding to the active site of HMG-CoA; this has been demonstrated by X-ray crystallography (Istvan and Deisenhofer 2001). Much has been made of the potential differences between the metabolism of the various statins and what makes the perfect statin, but the relative clinical impact of many of these factors is probably low apart from that of potential drug interactions, largely, but not fully, determined by differing metabolism through the cytochrome P450 system (Gaw *et al.* 2000; Betteridge and Khan 2003).

Lovastatin and simvastatin are administered as lactones which are metabolized to the open acid form in the liver whilst atorvastatin, fluvastatin, pravastatin, and rosuvastatin are administered as salts of their hydroxy acids. All statins are rapidly absorbed and reach peak concentrations at approximately 4–5hr. The degree of absorption varies, ranging from approximately 30 to 40% with atorvastatin, lovastatin, and pravastatin to rosuvastatin (50%), simvastatin and pitavastatin (80%), and fluvastatin (98%).

Statins undergo extensive first-pass metabolism by the liver and therefore have low systemic bioavailability and, apart from pravastatin (46–57%), are highly protein bound (88–99.5%). Most statins have a short elimination half-time (<2h) but the half-times of atorvastatin (11–30h) and rosuvastatin (19h) are considerably longer. Of the statins, pravastatin is the most hydrophilic compound followed by rosuvastatin; the others are lipophilic.

The liver is the site of metabolism of most statins. Atorvastatin, lovastatin, and simvastatin are metabolized through CYP 3A4 and fluvastatin is metabolized through CYP 2C9. Rosuvastatin undergoes only limited metabolism (10%) through CYP 2C9 and, to a lesser extent, 2C 19, and 90% is excreted unchanged in the faeces. Pravastatin is not metabolized through the CYP system and 60% is excreted in the urine (Gaw *et al.* 2000; Betteridge and Khan 2003). Clearly, there is potential for increased plasma levels if statin metabolism through CYP 450 enzymes is inhibited by other drugs. Of interest, grapefruit contains inhibitors of CYP 450 3A4 so should not be consumed to excess by patients taking simvastatin, lovastatin, and atorvastatin.

7.4 Clinical efficacy

Stains are highly effective, reducing LDL by 30–60% and are first-line therapy in the great majority of patients; those with polygenic hypercholesterolaemia, heterozygous familial hypercholesterolaemia, mixed lipaemia, familial combined hyperlipidaemia, and type 3 dyslipidaemia. Effects are dose dependent, independent of baseline LDL concentrations, and maximal after 3–4 weeks. Dose response is not linear; each doubling of dose results in an approximately 6% further reduction. Apoprotein B concentrations tend to be reduced to a similar degree to LDL. Effects on plasma triglycerides vary depending on baseline levels; with baseline triglycerides >2.8mmol/L, similar percentage reductions are seen to those for LDL, but when baseline levels are low effects on triglycerides are more modest (Stein *et al.* 1998). Effects on high-density lipoprotein (HDL) cholesterol are small, usually of the order of 5–10%.

Statins vary in their efficacy in reducing LDL, as shown in head-to-head comparative studies, the most effective being atorvastatin and rosuvastatin (Jones *et al.* 1998, 2003). Clearly efficacy is an important factor when choosing a particular drug, but other considerations include evidence of clinical benefit and safety in long-term RCTS, concomitant drug therapy, co-morbidities, appropriate treatment goals, and, increasingly, cost. This latter issue is largely determined by whether or not the particular drug is off patent.

7.5 **RCTs of statin therapy**

The Scandinavian Simvastatin Survival Study (4S) recruited patients with established coronary heart disease (CHD) (n = 4444, 827 females) and total cholesterol concentrations between 5.5 and 8.8mmol/L, despite dietary measures (The Scandinavian Simvastatin Survival Study Group 1994). Patients were randomized to simvastatin, 20–40mg/day or placebo. The primary end point was overall mortality, and the study needed to continue until 440 deaths had occurred to meet power calculations. In the simvastatin group, the treatment goal was a total cholesterol of 3.0–5.2mmol/L; 37% of patients required up-titration to 40mg/day.

LDL was reduced by 35%, and HDL increased by 8% compared to placebo. After a mean follow-up of 5.4yrs, 182 deaths occurred on simvastatin and 256 on placebo, a 30% reduction (HR 0.7; 95% CI 0.59–0.85; p < 0.0003). Major coronary events were reduced by 34%. Benefit was observed in women and in older as well as younger patients. Non-cardiac mortality and adverse events were similar to placebo. One case of rhabdomyolysis in the statin group recovered on drug cessation. The effects of 4S can be summarized as follows: more than 6yrs of simvastatin treatment of 100 CHD patients saved 4 deaths, 7 myocardial infarctions (MIs), and 6 revascularization procedures (The Scandinavian Simvastatin Survival Study Group 1994). Interestingly, in a further 8-yr follow-up of 4S there was continued survival benefit (Pedersen 2000).

Subsequent trials (see Table 7.2) have extended evidence for secondary prevention to patients with a wide range of baseline cholesterol levels (Sacks *et al.* 1996; LIPID Study Group 1998; Heart Protection Study Collaborative Group 2002; Serruys *et al.* 2002) irrespective of gender, age, baseline lipids, diabetes, metabolic syndrome, or hypertension. More recent trials comparing intensive statin therapy with standard therapy in stable coronary disease, together with studies in acute coronary syndromes, are discussed in Chapter 10.

The first primary prevention trial was the West of Scotland Coronary Prevention Study (WOSCOPS) (Shepherd *et al.* 1995) in which 6,595 men, aged 45–64yrs with LDL concentrations of 4.5–6mmo/L were randomized to placebo or pravastatin 40mg/day. Men with previous MI were excluded but those with stable angina were included so long as they had not been hospitalized in the preceding year. LDL was reduced by 26%, triglycerides was reduced by 12%, and HDL increased by 5%. The primary end point (coronary death and non-fatal MI) was reduced by 31% (95% CI, 17–43%; p < 0.001) after a mean follow-up of 4.9 years. Benefits were observed irrespective of baseline lipids, smoking status, age, or those with multiple risk factors. WOSCOPS can be summarized as follows: pravastatin treatment for 5yrs in 1,000 middle-aged men with hypercholesterolaemia saved 7 CVD deaths, 2 deaths from other causes, 20 non-fatal MIs, 8 revascularizations, and 14 angiograms (Shepherd et al. 1995).

Some might argue that WOSCOPS was not a true primary prevention trial in that some individuals had symptomatic angina; however, similar findings were described for a healthy population in the United States. A total of 6,605 subjects, 15% women, aged 55–73yrs with no clinical evidence of CVD were recruited on the basis of low HDL, <1.16mmo/L in men and <1.22mmol/L in women, and LDL concentrations of 3.36–4.91mmol/L in the Air Force/Texas Coronary Atherosclerosis Prevention Study (AFCAPS/TEXCAPS) (Downs et al. 1998) (see Table 7.1).

In the Anglo-Scandinavian Cardiac Outcomes Trial Lipid-lowering Arm (ASCOT-LLA), atorvastatin 10mg/day was compared with placebo in 10,305 hypertensive patients, aged 40–79yrs and random cholesterol ≤6.5mmol/L. The primary end point of fatal CHD and non-fatal MI after a median follow-up of 3.3yrs (the trial was stopped early on efficacy grounds) was reduced by 36% (0.64, 95% CI 0.50–0.83, p = 0.0005). Benefit was observed across all pre-specified subgroups and emerged in the first year of follow-up. An important observation in ASCOT-LLA was the 27% reduction in stroke with the statin in a population well treated for hypertension (Sever et al. 2003).

Although subgroup analyses of the major trials pointed to benefits in older patients, the Prospective Study of Pravastatin in the Elderly at Risk (PROSPER) trial provided efficacy and safety data in a specific elderly population (Shepherd et al. 2002). A total of 5,840 men and women aged 70–82yrs were recruited on the basis of previous coronary, cerebral, or peripheral vascular disease or increased CVD risk due to cigarette smoking, hypertension, or diabetes; baseline cholesterol levels were 4–9mmo/L and triglycerides <6mmol/L. Pravastatin (40mg/day) reduced LDL by 34% and, over a mean follow-up of 3.2yrs, the primary end point (coronary death, non-fatal MI, and fatal and non-fatal stroke) by 15% (0.85, 95% CI 0.74–0.97, p = 0.014) Surprisingly, there was no impact on stroke but the hazard ratio for transient ischaemic attack was 0.75 (5% CI 0.55–1.00, p = 0.051) (Shepherd et al. 2002).

Table 7.1 Primary prevention trials

Trial	Drug	Follow-up years	Primary end point	Event rate Placebo	Event rate Drug	Absolute risk reduction	Relative risk reduction	Significance
WOSCOPS	Pravastatin 40mg	4.9	Non-fatal MI, CHD death	248/3293 (7.9%)	174/3302 (5.5%)	2.4%	31%	P<0.001
AFCAPS/ TexCAPS	Lovastatin 20-40mg	5.2	Non-fatal MI, CHD death, unstable angina, sudden cardiac death	183/3301 (5.5%)	116/3304 (3.5%)	2.0%	37%	P<0.001
ASCOT-LLA	Atorvastatin 10mg	3.3	Non-fatal MI, CHD death	154/5137 (3%)	100/5168 (1.9%)	1.1%	36%	P<0.001
CARDS	Atorvastatin 10mg	3.9	Non-fatal MI, CHD death, unstable angina, resuscitated cardiac arrest, coronary revascularization, stroke	127/1410 (9.0%)	83/1428 (5.8%)	3.2%	37%	P<0.001

Table 7.2 Major secondary prevention trials								
Trial	Drug	Follow-up years	Primary end point	Event rate Placebo	Event rate Drug	Absolute risk reduction	Relative risk reduction	Significance
4S	Simvastatin 20–40mg	5.4	All cause mortality	256/2223 (11.5%)	182/2221 (8.2%)	3.3%	30%	P < 0.001
CARE	Pravastatin 40mg	5.0	Non-fatal MI,CHD death	274/2078 (13.2%)	212/2081 (10.2%)	3.0%	24%	p = 0.003
LIPID	Pravastatin 40mg	6.1	Non-fatal MI,CHD death	715/4502 (15.9%)	557/4512 (12.3%)	3.6%	24%	p < 0.001
HPS*	Simvastatin 40mg	5.0	All cause mortality	1507/10,267 (14.7%)	1328/10,269 (12.9%)	1.8%	13%	p < 0.001
*35% of patients had no prior coronary event			Fatal or non-fatal vascular events	2585/10,267 (25.2%)	2033/10,269 (19.8%)	5.4%	24%	p < 0.001

CHAPTER 7 **Pharmacological therapy**

Information on primary prevention in diabetes has come from the Heart Protection Study (HPS) (Heart Protection Study Collaborative Group 2003) and the Collaborative Atorvastatin Diabetes Study (CARDS) (Colhoun *et al.* 2004). HPS included 5,963 diabetic patients, aged 40–80yrs; 2,921 were free of vascular disease. In this group, simvastatin 40mg/day reduced first major vascular events by 33% (95% CI 17–46, p = 0.0003). After allowing for non-compliance the authors calculated that statin therapy would prevent about 45 people per 1,000 from having at least one major vascular event during the 5-yr treatment period. Benefits were seen irrespective of age, type, and duration of diabetes, hypertension, and pre-treatment cholesterol levels <5mmol/L (Heart Protection Study Collaborative Group 2003).

In CARDS, the first trial in a specific type 2 diabetic population, 2,838 patients, aged 40–75yrs with no previous history of CVD but with one other CVD risk factor (smoking, hypertension, albuminuria, or retinopathy) were randomized to atorvastatin 10mg or placebo (Colhoun *et al.* 2004). From a mean baseline of approximately 3mmol/L, statin therapy reduced LDL by 40% (1.2mmol/L), and this was associated with a 37% reduction (95% CI −52 to −17; p = 0.001) in first major CVD events. Mean duration of therapy was only 3.9 months, as the trial was terminated early after the second interim analysis. The authors calculated that atorvastatin would prevent at least 37 major vascular events per 1,000 patients treated for 4yrs (Colhoun *et al.* 2004).

The Cholesterol Treatment Trialists' (CTT) Collaborators have provided a meta-analysis of diabetic subjects (n = 18,686) included in the major studies, which strongly supports the evidence from HPS and CARDS (CTT Collaborators 2008). There were 3,247 major vascular events on which to base the analysis over a mean follow-up period of 4.3yrs. The analysis included 1,466 patients with type 1 diabetes amongst whom there were 343 major CVD events and 6165 women in whom there were 343 events. Effects on clinical outcomes were expressed per 1mmol/L reduction in LDL. Overall, there was a significant 9% reduction in overall mortality in those with diabetes which is similar to the 13% reduction in those without diabetes. The large database enabled subgroup analyses including those with type 1 diabetes; those with and without established CVD; women, age above or below 65yrs; normal or reduced estimated GFR and predicted vascular risk and similar benefits were observed (CTT Collaborators 2008).

7.6 **Safety**

Statins have proved to be safe and well tolerated. The reader is referred to some comprehensive reviews based on data from long-term RCTS and post-marketing surveillance (Pasternak *et al.* 2002; CTT Collaborators 2005; Grundy 2005; Davidson *et al.* 2006; Law *et al.* 2006). In the Cholesterol Trialists' Collaboration, statin therapy is not associated with an increase in non-cardiac deaths and the number of incident cancers is similar to placebo (CTT Collaborators 2005).

The reader is referred to the individual data sheets for the different compounds which list the various side effects, common ones being mild gastrointestinal effects, weakness, headaches, and aches and pains. Here the most serious adverse effects will be discussed, namely, myositis and liver function abnormalities.

Myositis, defined as generalized muscle pain and tenderness accompanied by a >10-fold increase in creatinine kinase concentration, which can progress to rhabdomyolysis and renal failure, is extremely rare. It is more frequent with higher doses but is not clearly related to the LDL-lowering. In a systematic review (Pasternak *et al.* 2002), estimated risk was 11 per 100,000 person years. This figure includes cases due to drug interactions. Even at high statin dose myositis is very rare, as, for instance, with atorvastatin, 80mg/day, based on 49 completed trials in 12,056 patients (Newman *et al.* 2006). In a large RCT of simvastatin 80mg/day there were 9 cases of myositis (de Lemos *et al.* 2004) and there does appear to be a step up in risk from 40mg/day as indicated in the data sheet. Less information is available for rosuvastatin because some long-term RCTS are awaited. However, in a recent study of 5,011 patients aged at least 60yrs with systolic heart failure, rosuvastatin 10mg/day did not produce an excess of myositis compared to placebo (Kjekshus *et al.* 2007). More safety data from an RCT will be available for rosuvastatin when the results of the JUPITER trial which has been terminated early because of benefits are published (www.brighamandwomens.org/preventive medicine/research/jupiter.aspx) expected late 2008. There is no evidence from RCTS that statins cause myalgia or muscle cramps (Armitage 2007).

A small percentage of patients develop abnormal liver function tests with raised transaminases. Whether these changes represent hepatotoxicity or are a result of LDL-lowering is not clear. Of interest, lipid-lowering with resins, which are not systemically absorbed can also increase transaminases. A greater than threefold rise is usually taken as significant. There is little evidence that these changes are associated with more serious liver damage, and they revert to normal on stopping the drug or reducing the dose (Armitage 2007). High transaminases are seen in 1–2% of patients on the 80 mg dose of atorvastatin (Newman *et al.* 2006). There is also a slight increase with simvastatin (de Lemos *et al.* 2004). Information from long-term RCTs provides the best information on adverse effects as there is no bias. Several possible adverse reactions including sleep and mood disorders, dementias, and peripheral neuropathy have been reported spontaneously but not seen in RCTs (Armitage 2007).

References

Armitage J (2007). The safety of statins in clinical practice. *The The Lancet*, **370**, 1782–90.

Betteridge DJ and Khan M (2003). *Statins and Coronary Artery Disease, 2nd edn.* Science Press Ltd, London.

Brown MS and Goldstein JL (1997). The SREBP pathway: regulation of cholesterol metabolism by proteolysis of a membrane-bound transcription factor. *Cell*, **89**, 331–40.

Cholesterol Treatment Trialists' (CTT) Collaborators (2005). Efficacy and safety of cholesterol-lowering treatment; prospective meta-analysis of data from 90.056 participants in 14 randomized trials of statins. *The Lancet*, **366**, 1267–78.

Cholesterol Treatment Trialists' (CTT) Collaborators (2008). Efficacy of cholesterol lowering therapy in 18,686 people with diabetes in 14 randomized trials of statins: a meta-analysis. *The Lancet*, **371**, 117–25.

Colhoun HM, Betteridge DJ, Durrington PN, *et al.* on behalf of the CARDS investigators (2004). Primary prevention of cardiovascular disease in type 2 diabetes in the Collaborative Atorvastatin Diabetes Study (CARDS): multicentre, randomized, placebo-controlled trial. *The Lancet*, **364**, 685–96.

Davidson MH, Clark JA, Glass LM, and Kanumalla A (2006). Statin safety: an appraisal from the adverse event reporting system. *The American Journal of Cardiology*, **97**, 32–43.

de Lemos JA, Blazing MA, Wiviott SD, *et al.* (2004). Early intensive versus a delayed conservative strategy in patients with acute coronary syndromes: phase Z of the Ato Z trial. *JAMA*, **292**, 1307–16.

Downs JR, Clearfield M, Weis S, *et al.*, for the AFCAPS/ TexCAPS Research Group (1998). Primary prevention of coronary events with lovastatin in men and women with average cholesterol levels: results of AFCAPS/TexCAPS. *JAMA*, **279**, 1615–22.

Endo A (1992). The discovery and development of HMG-CoA reductase inhibitors. *Journal of Lipid Research*, 33, 1569–82.

Gaw A, Packard CJ, Murray EF, *et al.* (1993). Effects of simvastatin on apoB metabolism and LDL subfraction distribution. *Arteriosclerosis Thrombosis*, **13**, 170–89.

Gaw A, Packard CJ, and Shepherd J (2000). *Statins: The HMG-CoA Reductase Inhibitors in Perspective.* Martin Dunitz, London.

Grundy SM (2005). The issue of statin safety: where do we stand? *Circulation*, **111**, 3016–19.

Heart Protection Study Collaborative Group (2002). MRC/BHF Heart Protection Study of cholesterol lowering with simvastatin in 20,536 high risk individuals: a randomized placebo-controlled trial. *The Lancet*, **360**, 7–22.

Heart Protection Study Collaborative Group (2003). MRC/BHF Heart Protection Study of cholesterol lowering with simvastatin in 5963 people with diabetes: a randomized placebo-controlled trial. *The Lancet*, **361**, 2005–16.

Istvan ES and Deisenhofer J (2001). Structural mechanism for statin inhibition of HMG-C0A reductase. *Science*, **292**, 1160–4.

Jones P, Davidson MH, Stein EA, *et al.* for the STELLAR Study Group (2003). Comparison of efficacy and safety of rosuvastatin versus atorvastatin, simvastatin, and pravastatin across doses (STELLAR Trial). *The American Journal of Cardiology*, **92**, 152–60.

Jones P, Kafonek S, Laurora I, *et al.* (1998). Comparative dose efficacy study of atorvastatin versus simvastatin, pravastatin, lovastatin and fluvastatin in patients with hypercholesterolaemia (the CURVES study). *The American Journal of Cardiology*, **81**, 582–7.

Kjekshus J, Apetrei E, Barrios V, *et al.* for the CORONA Group (2007). Rosuvastatin in older patients with systolic heart failure. *The New England Journal of Medicine*, **357**, 2248–61.

Law M and Rudnicka AR (2006). Statin safety: a systematic review. *The American Journal of Cardiology*, **97**, 52–60.

Long-Term Intervention with Pravastatin in Ischaemic Disease (LIPID) Study Group (1998). Prevention of cardiovascular events and death with pravastatin in patients with coronary heart disease and a broad range of initial cholesterol levels. *The New England Journal of Medicine*, **339**, 1349–57.

Newman CB, Palmer G, Silbershatz H, and Szarek M (2006). Comparative safety of atorvastatin 80 mg/day versus 10 mg/day derived from analysis of 49 completed trials in 12,056 patients. *The American Journal of Cardiology*, **97**, 61–7.

Pasternak RC, Smith SC Jr, Bairey-Merz CN, *et al.* (2002) ACC/AHA/NHLBI clinical advisory on the use and safety of statins. *Journal of the American College of Cardiology*, **40**, 567–72.

Pedersen TR, Wilhelmsen L, Faergeman O, *et al.* (2000). Follow-up study of patients randomised in the Scandinavian Simvastatin Survival Study (4S) of cholesterol lowering. *The American Journal of Cardiology*, **86**, 257–62.

Sacks FM, Pfeffer MA, Moye LA, *et al.* (1996). for the Cholesterol and Recurrent Events Trial Investigators. He effect of pravastatin on coronary events after myocardial infarction in patients with average cholesterol levels. *The New England Journal of Medicine*, **335**, 1001–9.

Serruys PW, de Freyter P, Macaya C, *et al.* for the Lescol Intervention. Prevention Study Investigators (2002). Fluvastatin for the prevention of cardiac events following successful first percutaneous coronary intervention: a randomized controlled trial. *JAMA*, **287**, 3215–22.

Sever PS, Dahlof B, Poulter NR, *et al.* for the ASCOT Investigators (2003). Prevention of coronary and stroke events with atorvastatin in hypertensive patients who have average or lower than average cholesterol concentrations in the Anglo-Scandinavian Cardiac Outcomes Trial-Lipid-Lowering Arm (ASCOT)-LLA): a multicentre randomized controlled trial. *The Lancet*, **361**, 1149–58.

Shepherd J, Blauw GJ, Murphy MB, *et al.* for the PROSPER Study Group (2002). Pravastatin in elderly individuals at risk of vascular disease (PROSPER): a randomized, controlled, trial. *The Lancet*, **360**, 1623–30.

Shepherd J, Cobbe SM, Ford I, *et al.* (1995). Prevention of coronary heart disease with pravastatin in men with hypercholesterolaemia in men with hypercholesterolaemia. *The New England Journal of Medicine*, **333**, 1301–7.

Stein EA, Lane M, and Laskarzewski P (1998). Comparison of statins in hypertriglyceridaemia. *The American Journal of Cardiology*, **81**, 66B–69B.

The Scandinavian Simvastatin Survival Study Group (1994). Randomised trial of cholesterol lowering in 4444 people with coronary heart disease: the Scandinavian simvastatin survival study (4S). *The Lancet*, **344**, 1383–9.

Vega GL, East C, and Grundy SM (1998). Lovastatin therapy in familial dysbetalipoproteinaemia: effects on kinetics of apolipoprotein B. *Atherosclerosis*, **70**, 131–43.

Chapter 8

Pharmacotherapy: non-statin drugs

D. John Betteridge

> **Key points**
>
> - Non-statin drugs do not have a large volume of data from randomized clinical trials (RCTs) to guide therapy but reasonable evidence exists for the fibrates, gemfibrozil, nicotinic acid, and the resins.
> - Non-statin drugs may be indicated in patients intolerant of statins or in whom statins are contraindicated.
> - Non-statin drugs may be added to statin therapy to obtain further effects on low-density lipoprotein (LDL) if treatment goals are not achieved on maximum-tolerated statin dose.
> - Non-statin drugs may be added to statin therapy to obtain further effects in increasing high-density lipoprotein (HDL) and reducing triglyceride.

8.1 Introduction

First choice drugs in the overwhelming majority of patients with dyslipidaemia are statins, but there are situations when the other drug classes provide either additional low-density lipoprotein (LDL)-lowering or complementary actions on other lipid and lipoprotein classes such as high-density lipoprotein (HDL)-cholesterol and triglycerides. Furthermore, despite their exceptional overall safety and tolerability, some patients do not tolerate statins. In this situation, knowledge of other drug classes and their potential benefits is clinically necessary for optimum patient management. All prescribers should consult data sheets of individual drugs before using them.

8.2 Fibrates

The first of these compounds, clofibrate (active metabolite chlorophenoxyisobutyrate) was developed more than 40yrs ago. This drug is now redundant as it caused gall stones through increased lithogenicity of bile and was of limited efficacy. Subsequently, there have been a series of more effective and better tolerated compounds.

8.2.1 **Mechanism of action**

Fibrates are agonists for peroxisome proliferator-activated receptor α (PPARα). PPARs are transcription factors that regulate gene expression in response to various natural ligands such as fatty acids. PPARα is expressed mainly in tissues that metabolize fatty acids such as liver, kidney, heart, and muscle. When activated, PPARα forms a heterodimer with retinoid X receptor (RXR) which binds to PPAR-specific response elements in the promoter regions of target genes. PPARs can also repress gene expression by interfering with other signalling pathways such as NF-κB, which is involved in inflammatory pathways (Schoonjans et al. 1996).

PPARα controls lipid and lipoprotein metabolism at different points. VLDL hydrolysis is stimulated through induction of lipoprotein lipase (LPL) and apoA-4, which enhances LPL activity, and by decreasing the expression of apoC-III, an inhibitor of the enzyme. PPARα has important effects on HDL metabolism through induction of apo-AI and apo-A2, the major apoproteins of HDL and the transport proteins ABCA1 (ATP-binding cassette A1) and SR-B1 (scavenger receptor class B1) involved in peripheral tissue cholesterol uptake by HDL and hepatic uptake respectively. Therefore, PPARα activation is likely to stimulate reverse cholesterol transport. Hepatic production of VLDL is decreased by PPARα activation of free fatty acid catabolism, thereby reducing the pool available for VLDL synthesis (Gervois et al. 2007).

8.2.2 **Clinical efficacy**

The main action of fibrates is to reduce plasma triglycerides and increase HDL. Triglyceride effects depend on baseline concentrations and reductions of 30–50% can be achieved. HDL can be increased by 5–15% depending on baseline concentrations and the particular lipid phenotype (Chapman 2003). The different fibrates tend to exert similar effects on triglycerides. Effects on LDL, however, do vary depending on the compound used and also on baseline levels and the lipid phenotype; effects are greater in pure hypercholesterolaemia than in mixed hyperlipidaemia. Least impact is seen with gemfibrozil (10%), then bezafibrate (15%), and then ciprofibrate and fenofibrate (20%). LDL subfraction distribution is altered with fibrate therapy towards larger, less dense particles. This probably explains the paradoxical increase in LDL when fibrates are used in isolated hypertriglyceridamia.

8.2.3 **RCTs of fibrate therapy**

The most consistent evidence is for gemfibrozil. The first fibrate, clofibrate, was used in the WHO Cooperative Trial, and it was the results of this trial that contributed to the cholesterol controversy of the 1980s and early 1990s. Clofibrate therapy which reduced cholesterol concentrations by 8% only (baseline 6.4mmol/L) in this large placebo-controlled trial (n = 10,000) over 5.3yrs was associated with a reduction of coronary events mainly because of a 25% reduction in non-fatal myocardial infarction (MI). This effect was overshadowed by an increase in non-coronary deaths. No particular cause of death predominated, but the lithogenic effect of clofibrate probably contributed to the excess of deaths in the 'liver, biliary, and intestines' category (Committee of Principal Investigators 1978). The design of the study has been subject to criticism particularly in the follow-up of out-of-trial mortality, and perhaps the most reliable data does relate to the effect on non-fatal MI. Nevertheless, clofibrate does cause gallstones and is redundant with the development of the second-generation drugs.

8.2.4 Gemfibrozil

Gemfibrozil has been used in two major RCTs. The Helsinki Heart Study (HHS), included 4,082 men, aged 40–55yrs, with baseline non-HDL-cholesterol ≥ 5.2mmol/L (baseline cholesterol: 6.9mmol/L) and no previous vascular disease. Gemfibrozil reduced LDL by 11%, reduced triglycerides by 35%, and increased HDL by 11%, and these changes were associated a 35% reduction (p <0.02) in the primary end point of fatal and non-fatal MI after a mean 5-year follow-up. There was no difference in overall deaths. Importantly, there was no significant increase in the rate of cholecystectomy (Frick *et al.* 1987). The authors reported that the benefit in HHS was partly related to the reduction in LDL and the increase in HDL and, in a *post hoc* analysis, a subgroup with an LDL/HDL cholesterol ratio >5 and a triglyceride >2.3mmol/L was identified as showing most benefit with a 71% reduction in coronary events (Manninen *et al.* 1992).

The Veterans Administration HDL Intervention Trial (VAHIT) tested the potential benefit of therapy to increase HDL in 2,531 men with established coronary disease and whose primary lipid abnormality was a low HDL. VAHIT included 25% of patients with a diagnosis of diabetes and 50% with the metabolic syndrome. Baseline lipid concentrations were LDL, 2.9mmol/L; triglycerides, 1.8mmol/L; and HDL, 0.8mmol/L. At one year HDL was increased 6% in the gemfibrozil (1.2g/day) group. Triglycerides were reduced by 31%, but there was no change in LDL. After a mean follow-up of 5.1yrs there was a 22% reduction in the primary end point (coronary death and non-fatal MI) of 22% (95% CI 7–35%, p = 0.006) (Rubins *et al.* 1999).

8.2.5 Bezafibrate

In the Bezafibrate Infarction Prevention (BIP) trial, 3,090 patients (2825 men) with previous MI or stable angina were randomized to bezafibrate, 400mg/day or placebo. Baseline lipid and lipoprotein concentrations were as follows: total cholesterol, 5.5mmol/L; LDL, 3.8mmol/L; HDL, 0.9mmol/L; and triglycerides, 1.6mmol/L. In the treatment group triglycerides were reduced by 17%, total cholesterol was reduced by 4.7%, LDL was reduced by 5.2%, and HDL increased by 14.4%. The primary end point was a composite of fatal and non-fatal MI and sudden death. Mean follow-up was 6.2 yrs, and the primary end point was reduced by 7.3%, which did not reach statistical significance. A *post hoc* analysis of patients with high baseline triglycerides (>2.26mmol/L) showed a 39.5% reduction in the primary end point (p = 0.02) (The BIP Study Group 2000). In a more recent analysis, patients fulfilling the criteria for metabolic syndrome showed benefit (Tenenbaum *et al.* 2005).

There has been speculation with regard to the discrepant results of VAHIT and BIP. Perhaps the difference is due to the different populations studied. For example, VAHIT included large numbers of patients with diabetes and the metabolic syndrome; 35% had a BMI >35 and 30% had insulin levels in the hyperinsulinaemia range. The event rate was higher in VAHIT, and drop in therapy with statin was low. In BIP there was 15% drop in the placebo group such that in the last 2yrs of the study there was a flattening of the Kaplan–Meier curves. Other possibilities include intrinsic differences between the drugs or the play of chance. It has been pointed out that the percentage of reduction in events in BIP falls within the 95% confidence intervals seen in VAHIT (Haffner 2000).

8.2.6 **Fenofibrate**

Given the impression that the fibrates were, if anything, more effective in metabolic syndrome and hypertriglyceridaemia, the outcome of the Fenofibrate Intervention and Event Lowering in Diabetes (FIELD) study was eagerly awaited (The FIELD Study Investigators 2005). In this combined primary and secondary CVD outcomes study in diabetic patients the primary end point (CHD death and non-fatal MI) did not reach statistical significance. Non-fatal MI was reduced significantly but coronary mortality showed a non-significant increase. Total cardiovascular events (cardiac death, MI, stroke, coronary, and carotid revascularization) were significantly reduced, but total mortality was non-significantly increased. The conflicting results of FIELD are puzzling. Baseline HDL in FIELD was 1.1mmol/L, whereas in VAHIT it was lower at 0.8mmol/L, and, perhaps, this lipid phenotype was better suited for intervention with the fibrate. In FIELD, fenofibrate had a disappointing long-term effect on HDL with barely a 2% increase by the end of the study. Furthermore, the reduction in LDL was only modest. Other confounders may be the adverse effect of fenofibrate in increasing homocysteine levels and higher drop in statin therapy in the placebo group. However, the major conclusion following the results of FIELD is that statins remain first-line therapy in diabetes (Colhoun 2005).

8.2.7 **Safety of fibrates**

The safety of fibrates is generally good. Side effects are generally mild; headache and gastrointestinal upsets are the most common complaints. Very rarely rashes and pruritis can occur. As with statins, myositis is extremely rare. In the FIELD study 3 patients on fenofibrate developed myositis compared to one on placebo, and 15 patients in the treated group compared to 10 controls showed creatinine phosphokinase (CPK) concentrations more than 5 times above normal (The FIELD Study Investigators 2005). Clofibrate undoubtedly precipitated gallstone formation in the WHO trial (59 vs 24 cholecystectomies) (Committee of Principal Investigators 1978), but this risk does not seem pronounced with newer agents (e.g., in HHS, 18 cholecystectomies vs 12, p = non-significant (NS)), but they are probably best avoided in patients with gall bladder disease. In FIELD there was a small but significant increase in pancreatitis which could reflect an increase in bile lithogenicity. There was a small excess of venous thrombolic events (The FIELD Study Investigators 2005).

In the author's opinion fibrates are best avoided in significant renal impairment as they can increase creatinine levels and the risk of side effects is increased. Careful monitoring of anticoagulants is necessary given their high protein binding. It is paradoxical that the fibrate with the best outcome data, gemfibrozil, should not be used with statins because it significantly increases blood levels and therefore the risk of myositis.

8.3 **Specific inhibitors of cholesterol absorption**

Ezetimibe is a novel, specific cholesterol absorption inhibitor which does not affect absorption of bile salts, triglycerides, or fat-soluble vitamins. It is available in a single-dose preparation of 10mg/day. It is also available in a combination tablet with simvastatin (Gagne et al. 2002).

8.3.1 **Mechanism of action**

Ezetimibe inhibits cholesterol absorption by approximately 50% in the proximal jejunum (Van Heek et al. 1997). The target of ezetimibe has been identified as Nieman-Pick C1-Like 1 (NPC1L1) in the brush border membranes of enterocytes (Garcia-Calvo 2005). Reduction of cholesterol absorption leads to reduction of cholesterol delivery to the liver, reduction in hepatic cholesterol content, up-regulation of LDL-receptors, and reduction of plasma LDL. This effect is partly offset because of an increase in hepatic cholesterol synthesis through activation of HMG-CoA reductase. This is the likely reason that the combination of ezetimibe with statins, inhibitors of the enzyme, is more than additive.

8.3.2 **Pharmacology and clinical efficacy**

Ezetimibe has a bioavailability of 35–65% and is rapidly glucuronidated and recycled by the enterohepatic circulation to its target site in the intestine. The metabolite is as potent as the parent compound in inhibiting cholesterol absorption. Both ezetimibe and its metabolite are highly protein bound and have half-lifes of 19–30hrs. Plasma concentration time plots show multiple peaks, suggesting enterohepatic recycling. The compound is primarily metabolized in the liver and small intestine by glucuronide conjugation; approximately 11% of the drug is excreted through the kidney, the bulk being excreted through the liver.

Ezetimibe reduces LDL concentrations by approximately 18%. Its effects can vary considerably between patients presumably related to the extent that they absorb cholesterol. When added to a statin there is a more than an additive effect with an additional LDL-lowering of 20–25%. Looked at simply, combination of ezetimibe with a statin at the lowest dose will lower LDL roughly the same as the top statin dose. For example, in patients with primary hypercholesterolaemia, baseline LDL, approximately 4.6mmol/L, ezetimibe alone lowered LDL by 18% and apoprotein B by 15%, but combined with atorvastatin across the dose range of 10–80mg/day, LDL reductions were 53%, 54%, 56%, and 61% (Ballantyne *et al.* 2003).

The co-administration of ezetimibe with fenofibrate has been studied in patients with mixed hyperlipidaemia (Farnier *et al.* 2005). Co-administration reduced LDL by 20.4%, non-HDL-cholesterol by 30.4%, and triglyceride by 44%, and increased HDL by 19%. And these effects were statistically significantly greater than either drug alone.

8.3.3 **Safety of ezetimibe**

This compound is generally very well tolerated (Forentin *et al.* 2008). Occasionally, there are gastrointestinal disturbances, headache and fatigue, myalgia, and rarely hypersensitivity reactions. When combined with statins, adverse events resemble those in statin monotherapy. Ezetimibe does not interact with drugs metabolized through the CYP P450 system and has no effect on bioavailability of warfarin. cyclosporin-A co-administration with ezetimibe results in an increase in exposure of ezetimibe of 2.3–12-fold (Bergman *et al.* 2006).

8.3.4 **RCTS of ezetimibe therapy**

There are as yet no long-term clinical end point studies reported with ezetimibe. However, there are ongoing studies. The Simvastatin and Ezetimibe in Aortic Stenosis (SEAS) study is evaluating the effects of the drug combination on CVD events and stenosis progression in patients with aortic stenosis (Rossebo *et al.* 2007). In the SHARP study (Study of Heart and Renal Protection) ezetimibe and simvastatin are being studied in a large number of patients with chronic kidney disease (Baigent and Landry 2003). The combination of simvastatin and ezetimibe is being compared with statin alone in acute coronary syndrome in the Improved Reduction of Outcomes: Vytorin Efficacy International Trial (www.schering-plough.com/pdf/IMPROVE.pdf).

8.4 **Nicotinic acid and derivatives**

The lipid-modifying effects of nicotinic acid are seen at high dose and are independent of its action as a vitamin (Altschul *et al.* 1955). The broad-spectrum effects of this drug in reducing LDL and triglycerides and substantially increasing HDL are highly attractive. However, its use has been limited by poor tolerability mainly related to the high incidence of cutaneous flushing. With the advent of statins, clinical attention has focussed on the potential of add-on nicotinic acid at lower dose to statins to reduce triglycerides and increase HDL-cholesterol. In addition, the tolerability of nicotinic acid has been improved by the development of extended-release (ER) forms and a blocker of the flush, laropiprant.

8.4.1 **Mechanism of action**

The mechanism(s) of action of nicotinic acid remain obscure (Walldius and Wahlberg 1999; Carlson 2005). Hepatic VLDL output is decreased, but the determinants of this effect remain to be fully explained. The drug reduces fatty acid release from adipose tissue, and this may decrease the uptake and incorporation of fatty acids into VLDL-triglyceride, which is also accompanied by reduced levels of cholesterol and apoprotein B. Other possible effects involve decreased de novo lipogenesis or esterification of fatty acids in the liver. Since LDL is the end product of the VLDL cascade, reduced VLDL will also result in reduced LDL. The increase in HDL appears to be due to reduced catabolism. Nicotinic acid can directly stimulate up-regulation of ATP-binding cassette transporter A1, a key modulator of reverse cholesterol transport in vitro (Rubic *et al.* 2004).

8.4.2 **Pharmacology and clinical efficacy**

The major usage of nicotinic acid in the statin era is the ER form at doses of 1–2g designed as add-on to statin therapy. Bioavailability of ER nicotinic acid is approximately 70% with a peak plasma concentration of 4hrs; it is less than 20% bound. It is metabolized through two pathways. The first involves the formation of nicotinamide adenine dinucleotide and nicotinamide, which is further metabolized to N-methylnicotinamide and to N-methyl-2-pyridone-5-carboxamide.

In the second pathway nicotinic acid is conjugated to glycine to form nicotinuric acid. At low doses the first pathway predominates and at higher doses it is saturated and unchanged nicotinic acid appears in the blood stream. The second pathway is not saturated across the relevant dose range. Nicotinic acid and its derivatives are rapidly eliminated in the urine.

ER nicotinic acid lowers triglycerides by approximately 35% and LDL by 16% and increases HDL by 25% at doses of 1–2g/day. LDL reduction is accompanied by a decrease in apoprotein B and the increase in HDL is accompanied by an increase in apoprotein A1 (Goldberg et al. 2000; McCormack and Keating 2005). Nicotinic acid is unique in that it will lower lipoprotein (a). In combination with statins there are marked effects on the overall lipid profile. ER nicotinic acid, 2g/day, and lovastatin, 40mg/day, was associated with reductions in triglycerides, LDL, and lipoprotein (a) of 41%, 45%, and 21%, respectively and an increase in HDL of 41% (Kashyap et al. 2002). Importantly, effects on HDL and triglycerides are significantly greater than statin alone together with the reduction of lipoprotein (a) (Bays et al. 2003).

8.4.3 **RCTs of nicotinic acid**

There is some RCT data for nicotinic acid. In the Coronary Drug Project (CDP) an early secondary prevention trial in men aged 30–64 yrs comparing different treatment strategies, nicotinic acid was the only therapy which significantly reduced the incidence of non-fatal MI (8.9% vs 12.2%, p <0.004). In a 9-yr follow-up of CDP previous nicotinic acid therapy was associated with an 11% reduction in mortality (p <0.004) (Canner et al. 1986). In an open-label study, a slow-release nicotinic acid preparation, niceritrol, and clofibrate in combination were compared with dietary treatment. Coronary death was reduced by 33% (47 vs 73, p <0.01) (Carlson and Rosenhamer 1988). In a subgroup analysis, those patients with a reduction in triglycerides of >30% showed most benefit. In addition, nicotinic acid has been used in combination therapy in several angiographic studies which have shown benefit on progression of atherosclerosis (Chapman 2005).

Ongoing trials with nicotinic acid such as the Treatment of HDL to Reduce the Incidence of Vascular Events (HPS-THRIVE, www.ctsu.ox.ac.uk) and the Atherosclerosis Intervention in Metabolic Syndrome with Low HDL-C/High Triglyceride and Impact on Global Health Outcomes study (AIM-HIGH, www.aimhigh.org) will provide further evidence on which to make treatment decisions.

8.4.4 **Safety of nicotinic acid**

Adverse reactions with the lower-dose ER preparation are much lower than with previous high doses of the crystalline form.

Gastrointestinal upsets, paraesthesia, pruritus, and erythema are observed in approximately 2% of patients. However, cutaneous flushing has been the main reason for drug discontinuation. This can be partly offset by starting at low dose with meals. The flush is prostaglandin mediated and is partly blocked by aspirin. Recently an ER preparation has been combined with laropiprant, a potent and selective antagonist of DP1, a G-protein-coupled receptor for prostaglandin D2 which mediates the flush. It is this combination which produces less flushing which is being studied in the HPS-THRIVE study.

Abnormal liver function tests (>3-fold aspartate aminotransferase (AST)) in about 1% of patients are generally asymptomatic and return to normal on drug cessation. Serious elevations in CPK (>10-fold) are seen in 0.3% of patients. There are many more laboratory and clinical adverse events that have been reported mainly with high doses, and the reader is directed to a comprehensive reviews (Goldberg et al. 2000; McCormack and Keating 2005). Importantly, the adverse effect of lower-dose ER nicotinic acid on glucose tolerance is much reduced compared to the high-dose crystalline form with increases in HbA1c of 0.1–0.2%. The American Diabetes Association advises that nicotinic acid at doses up to 2g/day can be used in patients with diabetes with appropriate monitoring and adjustment of therapy as necessary (American Diabetes Association 2004).

8.5 Resins

These drugs can be helpful in patients who are intolerant of statins. Two traditional resins are available in powder form, colestyramine, a copolymer of styrene and divinyl benzene, and colestipol, a copolymer of diethylpentamine and epichlorohydrin. Recently, a new, more powerful preparation, colesevalam hydrochloride, has become available in tablet form.

8.5.1 Mechanism of action

Resins act solely in the gut reducing the absorption of cholesterol and bile salt, thus interrupting the enterohepatic circulation (Hunninghake 1999). As a result, hepatic conversion of cholesterol to bile acids is increased through up-regulation of the rate-determining enzyme in bile-acid synthesis, 7α-hydroxylase. This leads to a reduction in hepatic cholesterol content, up-regulation of LDL-receptors, and consequently a decrease in plasma LDL. These effects are partly offset by increased hepatic cholesterol synthesis because of increased activity of HMG-CoA reductase.

8.5.2 **Clinical efficacy**

At moderate doses (colestyramine, 16g/day; colestipol, 20g/day) reductions in LDL of 15–30% are seen (Hunninghake, 1999). A small increase in HDL is often seen, but the mechanism of this effect is not understood. Plasma triglycerides may increase by 5–15%, possibly because of increased hepatic synthesis through activation of the enzyme, phosphatidate phosphohydrolase. This effect, more marked when baseline concentrations are raised, is usually transient. The resins are effective in both polygenic and heterozygous familial hypercholesterolaemia. Colesevelam, a more potent resin effective in tablet form, is associated with LDL reductions of around 15–19% at a dose of 3.75g/day (Bays and Dujovne 2003).

8.5.3 **RCTS of resins**

In the Lipid Research Clinics Coronary Primary Prevention Trial, 3806 men, aged 35–59yrs with a total cholesterol level greater than the 95th centile for the U.S. population, approximately 6.8mmol/L (baseline cholesterol 7.5mmol/L) received either colestyramine 24g/day or placebo. Study power was based on an assumption of a 25% difference in cholesterol but that achieved was only 9% because of compliance problems over the 7.4yrs of follow-up. Nevertheless there was a significant reduction in the primary end point (CHD death, non-fatal MI, and all-cause mortality), 155 events vs 187, p <0.05. There was no difference in overall mortality. Those individuals who took full-dose medication showed a 39.3% reduction in events and those who achieved an LDL reduction of 25% showed a 64% reduction in MI (Lipid Research Clinics Programme 1984).

8.5.4 **Safety of resins**

Statins are inconvenient to take, the powders need to be mixed with water, and the taste or the grittyness is tiresome. Main adverse effects relate to constipation, bloating, flatulence, heartburn, and nausea. These effects are partly offset by starting at low dose with gradual build-up and tend to ameliorate in time. Resins can interfere with the absorption of other drugs and should be taken at least 1h before or 4h after other medications. This can be a problem in patients on multiple therapies. High doses may interfere with the absorption of fat-soluble vitamins and supplementation may be required.

8.6 **Omega-3 fatty acids**

High-dose omega-3 fatty acid preparations have a role in the management of severe hypertriglyceridaemia. In the author's practice the preparation of preference is Omacor®, a highly purified preparation of eicosapentaenoic acid (EPA, 460mg) and docosahexaenoic acid (DHA 380mg) in a 1g capsule (Bays 2006). Each capsule contains vitamin E (4mg; 6 IU) as anti-oxidant. The preparation is extensively purified with undetectable levels of heavy metals, halogenated poly-carbons, and dioxins.

8.6.1 **Mechanism of action**

Omega-3 fatty acids are important regulators of many genes involved in lipid metabolism including PPARα and PPARγ. In addition, they inhibit the conversion of SREBP to its active form. Through these effects hepatic synthesis and output of triglycerides is likely to be reduced and LPL activity increased (Torrejon et al. 2007). Hepatic synthesis of triglycerides is also likely to be reduced because EPA and DHA are poor substrates for enzymes responsible for triglyceride synthesis.

8.6.2 **Pharmacology and clinical efficacy**

EPA and DHA as ethyl esters are absorbed orally and are incorpo-rated into phospholipid, although incorporation of DHA is less marked. In controlled clinical trials in patients with severe hypertrig-lyceridaemia (>5.65mmol/L), and mixed hyperlipidaemia, reductions in plasma triglycerides of 19–47% have been observed, the greater reductions being seen with higher baseline concentrations (Bays 2006). LDL concentrations are increased, but it is important to note that LDL levels are often low in severe hypertriglyceridaemia. Fur-thermore, there is a change in LDL subfraction distribution towards larger more buoyant particles. Effects on HDL vary with either no significant change or increases of up to 14% (Bays 2006; Torrejon et al. 2007).

8.6.3 **Safety of omega-3 fatty acids**

Omacor® is generally well tolerated and adverse reactions are rare. No adverse laboratory events have been described and no effects observed on plasma glucose levels. Prolongation of the bleeding time has been reported in some studies but not beyond the normal range. There is no interaction with drugs metabolized through the cytoch-rome P450 system.

8.6.4 **RCTs of omega-3 fatty acids**

There are no long-term clinical outcome trials using the dose of Omacor® (4g/day) for triglyceride-lowering. However, there is now considerable evidence of the benefits of omega-3 supplements on coronary events at doses not associated with significant lipid effects. In the Diet and Reinfarction Trial (DART), a secondary prevention trial, the consumption of oily fish twice weekly was associated with a 29% reduction in all-cause mortality (Burr et al. 1989). In a large secondary prevention trial, Omacor® (1g/day) was associated with a 30% reduction in cardiovascular death, a 45% reduction in sudden death and a 20% reduction in total mortality (GISSI Prevenzione

Investigators 1999). This finding is supported by several meta-analyses of other studies (Jacobson 2006) and is likely to be due to an anti-arrhythmic effect. A further CVD prevention trial, the Japan EPA Lipid Intervention Study (JELIS), used a purified preparation of EPA (1.8g/day) in patients (n = 18,645) already receiving statin therapy, the majority with no previous coronary disease. After 4.6yrs EPA therapy was associated with a reduction in the composite coronary heart disease end point of 19% (Yokoyama *et al.* 2007).

References

Altschul R, Hoffer A, and Stephen JD (1955). Influence of nicotinic acid on serum cholesterol in man. *Archives of Biochemistry and Biophysics*, **54**, 558–9.

American Diabetes Association (2004). Dyslipidaemia management in adults with diabetes. *Diabetes Care*, **27** (suppl 1), S68–71.

Baigent C and Landry M (2003). Study of heart and renal protection (SHARP). *Kidney International Supplement*, **84**, S207–10.

Ballantyne CM, Houri J, Notarbartolo A, et al. (2003). Effect of ezetimibe coadministered with atorvastatin in 628 patients with primary hypercholesterolaemia. A prospective, randomized, double-blind trial. *Circulation*, **107**, 2409–15.

Bays H (2006). Clinical overview of Omacor: a concentrated formulation of omega-3 polyunsaturated fatty acids. *American Journal of Cardiology*, **98** (suppl), 71i–6i.

Bays H and Dujovne C (2003). Colesevalam HCl: anon systemic lipid-altering drug. *Expert Opinion in Pharmacotherapy*, **4**, 779–90.

Bays HE, Dujovne CA, McGovern ME, et al. (2003). Comparison of once-daily niacin extended-release/lovastatin with standard doses of atorvastatin and simvastatin. *American Journal of Cardiology*, **91**, 667–72.

Bergman AJ, Burke J, Larson P, et al. (2006). Interaction of single-dose ezetimibe and steady-state cyclosporine in renal transplant patients. *Journal of Clinical Pharmacology*, **46**, 328–36.

Burr ML, Fehily AM, Gilbert JF, et al. (1989). Effects of changes in fat, fish and fibre intakes on death and myocardial reinfarction: diet and reinfarction trial (DART). *The Lancet*, **2**, 757–61.

Canner PL, Berge KG, Wenger NK, et al. (1986). Fifteen year mortality in coronary drug project patients: long-term benefit withniacin. *JACC*, **8**, 1245–55.

Carlson LA (2005). Nicotinic acid: the broad-spectrum lipid drug. A 50th anniversary review. *Journal of Internal Medicine*, **258**, 94–114.

Carlson LA and Rosenhamer G (1988). Reduction of mortality in the Stockholm ischaemic heart disease secondary prevention study by combined treatment with clofibrate and nicotinic acid. *Acta Medica Scandinavica*, **223**, 405–18.

Chapman MJ (2003). Fibrates in 2003: therapeutic action in atherogenic dyslipidaemia and future perspectives. *Atherosclerosis*, **171**, 1–13.

Chapman MJ (2005). The potential role of HDL and LDL-cholesterol modulation in atheromatous plaque development. *Current Medical Research and Opinion*, **21** (suppl 6), S17–22.

Colhoun H (2005). After FIELD: should fibrates be used to prevent cardiovascular disease in diabetes? *The Lancet*, **366**, 1829–31.

Committee of Principal Investigators (1978). Report on a cooperative trial in the primary prevention of ischaemic heart disease using clofibrate. *British Heart Journal*, **40**, 1069–118.

Farnier M, Freeman MW, Macdonell G, et al. (2005). Efficacy and safety of the coadministration of ezetimibe with fenofibrate in patients with mixed hyperlipidaemia. *European Heart Journal*, **26**, 897–905.

Forentin M, Liberopoulos EN, and Elisaf MS (2008). Ezetimibe-associated adverse effects: what the clinician needs to know. *International Journal of Clinical Practice*, **62**, 88–96.

Frick MH, Elo O, Haapa K, et al. (1987). The Helsinki Heart Study: primary prevention trial with gemfibrozil in middle-aged men with dyslipidaemia. Safety of treatment, changes in risk factors and incidence of coronary heart disease. *The New England Journal of Medicine*, **317**, 1237–45.

Gagne C, Bays H, Weiss S, et al. (2002). Efficacy and safety of ezetimibe added to ongoing statin therapy for treatment of patients with primary hypercholesterolaemia, *American Journal of Cardiology*, **90**, 1084–91.

Garcia-Calvo M, Lisnock J-M, Bull HG, et al. (2005). The target of ezetimibe is Niemann-Pick C1-Like 1 (NPC1L1). *PNAS*, **102**, 8132–7.

Gervois P, Fruchart J-C, and Staels B (2007). Drug Insight: mechanisms of action and therapeutic applications for agonists of peroxisome proliferator-activated receptors. *Nature Clinical Practice Endocrinology and Metabolism*, **3**, 145–56.

GISSI Prevenzione Investigators (1999). Dietary supplementation with n-3 polyunsaturated fatty acids and vitamin E after myocardial infarction: results of the GISSI-Prevenzione Trial. *The Lancet*, **354**, 447–55.

Goldberg A, Alagona P Jr., CapuzziDM, et al. (2000). Multiple-dose efficacy and safety of an extended-release form of nicotinic acid in the management of hyperlipidaemia. *American Journal of Cardiology*, **85**,1100–5.

Haffner SM (2000). Secondary prevention of coronary heart disease. The role of fibric acids. *Circulation*, **102**, 2–4.

Hunninghake DB (1999). Bile-acid sequestering agents (resins). In Betteridge DJ, Illingworth DR, and Shepherd J, eds. *Lipoproteins in Health and Disease*, pp 1133–44. Arnold, London.

Jacobson TA (2006). Secondary prevention of coronary artery disease with omega-3 fatty acids. *American Journal of Cardiology*, **98** (suppl), 61i–70i.

Kashyap ML, McGovern ME, Berra K, et al. (2002). Long-term safety and efficacy of a once-daily niacin/lovastatin formulation forpatients with dyslipidaemia. *American Journal of Cardiology*, **89**, 672–8.

Lipid Research Clinics Programme (1984). The Lipid Research Clinics Coronary Primary Prevention Trial Results. 1. Reduction in incidence of coronary heart disease, *JAMA*, **251**, 351–64.

Manninen V, Tenkanen H, Koskinen P, et al. (1992). Joint effects of trigly-cerides and LDL-cholesterol and HDL-cholesterol concentrations on coronary heart disease risk in the Helsinki Heart Study. Implications for treatment. *Circulation*, **85**, 37–45.

McCormack PL and Keating GM (2005). Prolonged-released nicotinic acid. A review of its use in the treatment of dyslipidaemias. *Drugs*, **65**, 2719–40.

Rossebo AB, Pedersen TR, Allen C, et al. (2007). Design and baseline characteristics of the simvastatin and ezetimibe in aortic stenosis (SEAS) study. *American Journal of Cardiology*, **99**, 970–3.

Rubic T, Trottman M, and Lorenz RL (2004). Stimulation of CD36 and the key effector of reverse cholesterol transport ATP- binding cassette A1 in monocytoid cells by niacin. *Biochemical Pharmacology*, **67**, 411–9.

Rubins HB, Robins SJ, Collins D, et al. (1999). Gemfibozil for the second-ary prevention of cronary heart disease in men with low levels of high density lipoprotein cholesterol. *The New England Journal of Medicine*, **341**, 410–18.

Schoonjans K, Staels B, and Auwerx J (1996). The peroxisome proliferator activated receptors (PPARs) and their effects on lipid metabolism and adipocyte differentiation. *Biochimica et Biophysica Acta*, **1302**, 93–109.

Tenenbaum A, Motro M, Fisman EZ, et al. (2005). Bezafibrate for the secondary prevention of myocardial infarction in patients with metabolic syndrome. *Archives of Internal Medicine*, **165**, 1154–60.

The BIP Study Group (2000). Secondary prevention by raising HDL-cholesterol and reducing triglycerides in patients with coronary artery disease: the Bezafibrate Infarction Prevention (BIP) Study. *Circulation*, **102**, 21–7.

The FIELD Study Investigators (2005). Effects of long-term fenofibrate therapy on cardiovascular events in 9795 people with type 2 diabetes mellitus (the FIELD study): randomized controlled trial. *Lancet*, **366**, 1849–61.

Torrejon C, Jung UJ, and Deckelbaum RJ (2007). n-3 fatty acids and cardi-ovascular disease: actions and molecular mechanisms. *Prostaglandins, Leukotrienes and Essential Fatty Acids*, **77** (5–6), 319–26.

Van Heek M, France C, Compton D, et al. (1997). In vivo metabolism-based discovery of a potent cholesterol absorption inhibitor, SCH 58235, in the rat and rhesus monkey through the identification of active metabolites of SCH 48461. *The Journal of Pharmacology and Experimental Therapeutics*, **283**, 157–63.

Walldius G and Wahlberg G. (1999). Nicotinic acid and its derivatives. In Betteridge DJ, Illingworth DR, and Shepherd J, eds. *Lipoproteins in Health and Disease,* pp. 1181–97. Arnold, London.

Yokoyama M, Origasa H, Matsuzaki M, et al. (2007). Effects of eicosapen-taenoic acid (EPA) on major coronary events in hypercholesterolaemic patients (JELIS): a randomised open-label blinded end point analysis. *Lancet*, **369**, 1090–8.

Chapter 9

Combination therapy for the management of hyperlipidaemia

Anthony S. Wierzbicki

Key points

- Low doses of multiple drugs can be combined to treat patients intolerant to statin therapy
- Combination therapy to reduce LDL-C is increasingly necessary to reduce LDL-C > 50% as required in the highest risk patients
- Statins have little effect on risk driven by low HDL-C and increasingly niacin (nicotinic acid) and fibrates are used in combination with statins to optimize the total lipid profile
- Large-scale end point studies with statin-other drug combinations are underway.

9.1 Introduction

Statin therapy is well established in all guidelines as the first line treatment for all patients with or at risk of developing cardiovascular disease. As shown in the Cholesterol Treatment Triallists' Collaboration statin therapy is associated with a 12% reduction in mortality and a 22% reduction in cardiovascular events per 1mmol/L LDL-C reduction. However, not all patients tolerate statin therapy at the doses necessary to produce 1mmol/L or >30% LDL-C reductions thought necessary in modern practice. In addition patients at very high of recurrent events require more aggressive LDL-C reduction with decrements of 50% being shown to be necessary in acute coronary syndromes and in patients with stable coronary heart disease in trials such as PROVE-IT, TnT, and IDEAL. Thus, increasingly combination therapy is necessary to achieve the necessary LDL-C reductions in these patients. While statins are excellent drugs in reducing the risk of atherosclerosis associated with LDL-C they have only minimal effects on HDL-C and a substantial residual risk remains in patients with low levels of this protective lipid sub-fraction. Thus there is an opportunity to combine statins with drugs that raise HDL-C such as fibrates or niacin (nicotinic acid).

9.2 **Combination therapy in the statin intolerant**

Statins are a relatively novel development in the field of lipid lowering and older drugs such as bile acid sequestrants, fibrates and nicotinic acid have been shown to reduce cardiovascular events in trials such as the Lipid Research Clinics (colestyramine; 19%), Helsinki Heart Study and Veterans Affairs HDL Intervention Trial (gemfibrozil; 23–34%) and the Coronary Drug Project (niacin (nicotinic acid); 23%). Ezetimibe is a specific inhibitor of the duodenal NPC1L1 cholesterol transporter and produces a 15–20% reduction in LDL-C but has as yet has no endpoint evidence. All of these drugs reduce LDL-C.

Statin intolerance is both idiosyncratic and dose/drug strength-related. Patients who are statin intolerant may have autoimmune or genetic muscle disease, be hypothyroid, or have low muscle mass and impaired renal function. In general any statin trialled at ultra-high (unlicensed) doses (e.g., simvastatin 160mg or rosuvastatin 80mg) to produce a >50% LDL-C reduction is associated with an excess of gastrointestinal or myopathic side effects. In some individuals these effects occur at far lower doses limiting the use of statin therapy. In these patients recourse is made to low dose statin + ezetimibe (see below) in the first instance but the truly intolerant require alternative approaches. The exact choice of agent depends on the patient but most commonly halogenated fibrates (that reduce LDL-C by 9–25%, e.g. fenofibrate) are combined with ezetimibe to deliver a 25–30% reduction in LDL-C. Fibrates, like statins, can cause myalgia so in these patients with a very low threshold for muscle side effects niacin (nicotinic acid) is often substituted as this agent has an even lower rate of muscle side effects as nicotinic acid reduces LDL-C by up to 25% with 2g/day but at the price of an increase of prostaglandin D_2 induced flushing which can be partially ameliorated with aspirin therapy. A novel formulation of niacin with a prostaglandin D_2 type 1 receptor blocker (MK-0524; laropiprant) is in development and may offer superior tolerability. In the truly systemic therapy intolerant resort can be made to a combination of ezetimibe and a bile acid sequestrant. The older bile acid sequestrants (colestyramine, colestipol) are associated with a 30–40% incidence of nausea, bloating and gastrointestinal side effects. Newer non-ionic bile acid sequestrants e.g. colesevelam are associated with lower rates of side effects (10%).

This combination can be effective if correctly temporally spaced (as ezetimibe is bound by bile acid sequestrants) as the two drugs target different points in the cholesterol absorption pathway—the duodenum and terminal ileum—and thus deliver additive effects.

9.3 **Combination therapy to reduce LDL-C**

Though statins are commonly recommended to be used at a dose likely to produce >1mmol/L reduction in LDL-C (e.g., simvastatin or pravastatin 40mg) there is now evidence that even low doses (e.g. pravastatin 10mg) can produce reductions in cardiovascular events after a reduction in LDL-C of 20%. In the low risk primary prevention population studied in ther MEGA study with a LDL-C of 4.5 mmol/L, pravastatin therapy was associated with a 42% reduction in cardiovascular events after 5yrs. In patients unable to tolerate daily statin these drugs are sometimes used on alternate days or even for long half-life agents (e.g., rosuvastatin 5mg) weekly. As these low doses give reductions in LDL-C of 10–20% it is necessary to combine them with other compounds.

The commonest combination is the use of a statin with ezetimibe as this combination is associated with an effective reduction of the statin dose by three dose increments as each doubling of statin dose delivers an extra 5–7% LDL-C reduction. The mechanism by which this works is that statin therapy not only increases hepatocyte LDL-receptor expression but also upregulation of HMG-CoA reductase production and also intestinal cholesterol absorption. Thus addition of a cholesterol uptake blocker delivers an additive effect on LDL-C in the vast majority of patients. The combination is also well tolerated with a side-effect rate in the region of 2%—mostly due to gastrointestinal side effects and can deliver a 60–70% reduction in LDL-C levels at the highest licensed doses.The use of statin-ezetimibe has largely superseded the use of bile acid sequestrants (resins) as these drugs are associated with a 30–40% incidence of nausea, bloating and gastrointestinal side effects. Newer non-ionic bile acid sequestrants e.g. colesevelam are associated with lower rates of side effects (10%). Endpoint trial evidence on the combination of statins with ezetimibe will come from studies in patients with aortic stenosis (SEAS), chronic renal failure (SHARP) and in acute coronary syndromes (IMPROVE-IT) in the next few years.

However, despite statin-ezetimibe resulting in attainment of the new National Cholesterol Education Program or other guideline goals in 80–90% of patients some individuals show a degree of statin resistance. This arises through a number of mechanisms including changes in expression of the organic anion transporter necessary for statin acid uptake, induction of drug pumps (e.g., P-glycoprotein/

MDR-2 protein) but also increased expression of HMG-CoA reductase such that in some patients mevalonic acid (the post HMG-Co reductase intermediate in cholesterol synthesis) can be detected in the plasma of patients after 6–12hrs. Thus additional methods are required to reduce LDL-C in these patients. A number of compounds are in development to target either the cholesterol synthesis or lipoprotein assembly pathways. The cholesterol synthesis pathway can additionally be blocked at squalene synthase and lapaquisat (TAK-475) is in phase 3 clinical trials as an additive therapy to statins. This agent delivers an additional 20–25% LDL-C reduction in monotherapy or added to statins and may have the additional advantage of raising the levels of isoprenoid intermediates and thus reducing the incidence of myalgia if this occurs through mitochondrial deficiency of ubiquinone (Co-enzyme Q-10). More radical approaches involve disrupting the assembly of very-low density lipoprotein (VLDL) in the liver. This can be performed either through subcutaneous injection of an antisense RNA to apolipoprotein B-100 as shown in clinical trials of ISIS-302101 or by inhibition of microsomal transfer protein that adds triglycerides and cholesterol to nascent VLDL. In contrast to antisense therapy, inhibition of MTP induces hepatic steatosis so trials of MTPIs are exploring progressively lower doses of these compounds that still maintain efficacy in delivering a >20% reduction in LDL-C.

9.4 **Combination therapy to reduce LDL-C and raise HDL-C**

As the epidemiology of atherosclerosis changes in parallel with the vast rates of increase in obesity, the metabolic syndrome and type 2 diabetes, the typical lipid profile is changing. The pure hypercholesterolaemia (Fredricksen 2a) often seen 20yrs ago is less common and increasingly mixed hyperlipidaemia (type 2b-4) is found with the typical profile of reduced HDL-C and raised triglycerides of the metabolic syndrome or type 2 diabetes. Statins are effective in reducing cardiovascular risk in direct proportion to the underlying risk level and reduce triglycerides both as a function of their own potency and of baseline triglyceride levels.Their effects on HDL-C are variable and dose dependent ranging from neutral to slightly positive (up to 14%). Data from the statin trials shows that they have no effect on HDL-C driven risk so patients with low HDL-C treated with statins have higher subsequent event rates than placebo groups with high HDL-C. Thus, there is an increasing emphasis on combing drugs to raise HDL-C with statin therapies.

There are many ways to raise HDL-C including exercise, weight reduction, and treatment of hyperglycaemia with insulin or some thiazolidinediones. Many of these treatment modalities can be easily combined with statin therapy. In terms of specific lipid lowering drugs there is some evidence that combination therapy can reduce progression of coronary or carotid atherosclerosis. The Stockholm Ischaemic Heart Disease Study showed a 36% reduction in coronary heart disease events in an underpowered study that compared the combination of clofibrate and niacin (nicotinic acid) with placebo. Clofibrate has been discontinued as newer fibrates that cause less gallstone formation and are not associated with excess mortality have become available. A number of studies have combined fibrates (usually gemfibrozil) with nicotinic acid and colestyramine and shown a reduction in coronary atherosclerosis progression (e.g., Air Force Regression Study; AFREGS). Other studies have combined statins (usually low dose) with nicotinic acid and colestyramine again examining coronary artery disease progression. In the 15-year follow-up of the Familial Atherosclerosis Trial triple combination therapy was associated with a 75% reduction in events. In the HDL Atherosclerosis Therapy Study (HATS), niacin (nicotinic acid) combined with moderate dose statin was again associated with a reduction in coronary progression and a similar reduction in events while in the small ARBITER-2 study low dose niacin (nicotinic acid) with high-dose statin therapy resulted in a reduction in progression of carotid intima-media thickness. These trials typically show reductions in LDL-C of 40–50%; triglycerides by 30–40% and rises in HDL-C of 20–25%. End point trials combining nicotinic acid (with/without laropiprant) with optimal statin and ezetimibe therapy are now underway in secondary prevention patients with atherogenic dyslipidaemia (AIM-HIGH; n=3,300) or patients at high risk of cardiovascular disease (HPS-2; THRIVE; n=20,000) based on the premise of additive action for these combinations.

The role of statin-fibrate combination therapy is less clear. Much of the problem arises from safety concerns and the conflicting clinical trial data on the efficacy of fibrates though recent meta-analyses suggest a benefit on non-fatal myocardial infarction with these drugs. The combination of statins metabolized through cytochrome P450 3A4 (lovastatin, simvastatin, atorvastatin) with gemfibrozil is associated with a 5-fold increase in the rate of rhabdomyolysis. In the case of cerivastatin the increase was 50-fold and caused the withdrawal of ther drug. The mechanism of the interaction relates to the inhibition of glucuronidation of statin acids (the active moieties) by gemfibrozil. In contrast both fenofibrate and bezafibrate seem to have low levels of excess rhabdomyolysis (2-fold) when combined with statins. Cohort studies show that fibrate-statin therapy is effective in delivering long-term reductions in LDL-C (30–40%) and triglycerides (30–50%) and in raising HDL-C by 20–25% and in one retrospective cohort study may reduce events in proportion to the degree of triglyceride reduction. The only significant prospective endpoint clinical trial data on the combination is the statin drop-in sub-group in the FIELD study of patients with early type 2 diabetes. This is difficult to interpret as not only was no benefit seem, the lipid changes were not typical of combination therapy. The large scale ACCORD trial of fenofibrate and simvastatin 40mg in patients with type 2 diabetes (n=5,800) may answer the questions about the efficacy of statin-fibrate combination therapy.

9.5 **Combination therapy for hypertriglceyeridaemia**

The mainstays of treatment for hypertriglyceridaemia are fibrates. These are used extensively for patients with triglycerides >4.7mmol/L or >1.7–2.3mmol/L in patients with diabetes usually in addition to primary statin therapy. In type 4 and type 5 hyperlipidaemia where triglycerides are >10mmol/L and >20mmol/L fibrates are used first line and reduce triglycerides by 40–60%. However often this is insufficient to fully control the hyperlipidaemia and a resort has to be made to combination therapy to reduce risks of pancreatitis and subsequent beta-cell failure induced type 2 diabetes which will exacerbate any underlying hypertriglyceridaemia. There is little trial evidence in this field but common combinations used are fibrate with high-dose omega-3 fatty acids, fibrate-nicotinic acid and increasingly fibrate–statin. Fibrates in combination with statins increase lipoprotein lipase production and decrease apolipoprotein-C3 (a triglyceride-rich remnant uptake inhibitory protein) and increase LDL-receptor levels and so increase clearance mostly probably through apolipoprotein E dependent pathways. Fibrate-statin therapy can deliver an 80% reduction in triglycerides, and a 50% increase in HDL-C in these patients and almost normalise the lipid profile.

9.6 **Conclusions**

Statins are now accepted as first line therapy for the vast majority of hyperlipidaemia but as LDL-C targets are progressively reduced for the highest risk patients increasing recourse is having to be made to combination therapy to deliver LDL-C goals. Similarly as the critical role of low HDL-C in the progression of coronary heart disease is recognised it is becoming necessary to combine statins with HDL-C raising therapies. It is likely that as optimization of complete lipid profiles is viewed as essential, the management of hyperlipidaemia will become very similar to the management of hypertension or diabetes where multiple drugs with complementary mechanisms of action are used to reduce cardiovascular risk.

References

Baigent C, Keech A, Kearney PM, *et al.* (2005). Efficacy and safety of cholesterol-lowering treatment: prospective meta-analysis of data from 90,056 participants in 14 randomised trials of statins. *The Lancet*, **366**, 1267–78.

Wierzbicki AS, Mikhailidis DP, Wray R, *et al.* (2002). Statin-fibrate combination therapy for hyperlipidaemia :a review. *Current Medical Research and Opinion*, **19**, 155–68.

Wierzbicki AS (2004). Lipid-altering agents: the future. *International Journal of Clinical Practice*, **58**, 1063–72.

Wierzbicki AS (2006a). FIELDS of dreams, fields of tears: a perspective on the fibrate trials. *International Journal of Clinical Practice*, **60**, 442–9.

Wierzbicki AS (2006b). Future approaches to reducing low-density lipoprotein cholesterol. *Future Lipidology*, **1**, 463–77.

Wierzbicki AS (2006c). Low HDL-cholesterol: Common and under-treated, but which drug to use? *International Journal of Clinical Practice*, **60**, 1149–53.

Chapter 10

Recent lipid-lowering trials in perspective: implications for therapy

D. John Betteridge

Key points

- Despite the clinical benefits of statin therapy in primary and secondary cardiovascular disease (CVD) prevention trials, considerable residual risk persists.
- Meta-analysis of major randomized controlled trials (RCTs) suggests that greater low-density lipoprotein (LDL)-lowering is associated with greater reduction in events.
- Recent RCTs in stable coronary disease and in acute coronary syndrome have demonstrated greater benefit with more intensive LDL-lowering.
- The results of these trials have changed LDL goals of therapy for those at highest risk.

10.1 Introduction

Early lipid-lowering trials with statins and other agents have been discussed in Chapters 7 and 8. In this chapter, more recent trials on the potential benefits of more intensive low-density lipoprotein (LDL)-cholesterol-lowering in coronary disease will be discussed given the implications for treatment targets in high-risk individuals.

10.2 The Cholesterol Trialists' Collaboration

The Cholesterol Trialists' Collaboration (CTT), a meta-analysis of 14 randomized statin trials involving 90,056 participants, provided impressive evidence of the benefits and the safety of statin therapy (CTT Collaboration 2005). In this large database, there were a total of 8,186 deaths, 14,348 individuals with major vascular events, and

5,103 individuals with cancer on which to analyse benefits and risk. The difference in LDL achieved in these trials ranged from 0.35mmol/L to 1.77mmol/L at 1yr. The authors calculated that an LDL reduction of 1mmol/L is associated with a 12% reduction in all-cause mortality [rate ratio (RR) 0.88, 95% confidence interval (CI) 0.84–0.91; $p < 0.0001$] and a 19% reduction in coronary mortality (0.81, 0.76–0.85; $p < 0.0001$). As expected, there were important reductions in non-fatal vascular events. The benefits observed were independent of previous vascular disease, age and sex, presence of hypertension or diabetes, and baseline lipids (CTT Collaboration 2005). Benefits were observed at 1yr and became greater in subsequent years. The authors calculated that the overall reduction of about one-fifth in major vascular events per mmol/L LDL-cholesterol reduction would translate into 48 fewer individuals with previous disease developing events per 1,000 treated and 25 fewer with no previous disease. Cancers were identical between the treated and placebo groups.

An important, but perhaps predictable, finding from CTT is that the proportional reduction in major vascular events is strongly related to the absolute LDL reduction achieved (CTT Collaboration 2005). This finding has received considerable support from recent randomized controlled trials (RCTs) in patients with stable coronary disease and in acute coronary syndromes (ACS).

10.3 **Intensive versus standard statin therapy**

In the treat to new targets (TNT) trial, intensive statin therapy (atorvastatin 80mg/day) was compared to standard therapy (atorvastatin 10mg/day) in patients with stable coronary disease (LaRosa *et al.* 2005). Men and women (n=15,464), aged 35–75yrs with previous coronary disease and LDL concentrations of 3.4–6.5mmol/L entered an 8-week treatment run-in period with atorvastatin 10mg/day. Those individuals who achieved a mean LDL <3.4mmol/L (n=10.001) were randomized to double-blind therapy with either atorvastatin 10mg/day or 80mg/day for a median of 4.9yrs. Mean LDL was 2.0mmol/L on treatment with atorvastatin 80mg/day compared to 2.6mmol/L on atorvastatin 10mg/day. Primary end points, a composite of coronary death, non-fatal myocardial infarction (MI), resuscitated cardiac arrest, or fatal or non-fatal stroke occurred in 434 patients (8.7%) on the 80mg dose compared to 548 patients (10.9%) on the 10mg dose [hazard ratio (HR) 0.78, 95% CI 0.69–0.89; $p < 0.001$].

Given the high risk of diabetic patients with coronary heart disease (CHD), the results from the diabetic subgroup (n=1,501) analysis of TNT are important. Mean LDL-cholesterol in the intensive therapy group was 2.0mmol/L compared to 2.5mmol/L in the standard therapy group and this was associated with a 25% risk reduction in major cardiovascular events (HR 0.75, 95% CI 0.58–0.97; p = 0.026) (Shepherd et al. 2006).

The IDEAL study (Incremental Decrease in End Points Through Aggressive Lipid-Lowering) asked a similar question but compared two different drug regimens, simvastatin 20–40mg/day and atorvastatin 80mg/day, and the results were less clear cut but certainly compatible with the results of TNT (Pedersen et al. 2005). A total of 8,888 CHD patients (age <80yrs) were randomly allocated to simvastatin 20–40mg/day (achieved LDL, 2.7mmol/L) or atorvastatin 80mg/day (achieved LDL, 2.1mmol/L). The trial was open-label but with blinded end-point evaluation, the so-called PROBE design. After a median follow-up of 4.8yrs, there was a non-significant reduction in the primary end point (a composite of coronary death, non-fatal MI, or resuscitated cardiac arrest) of 11% (0.89; 95% CI 0.78–1.01; p = 0.07). A post hoc Cox regression analysis of the primary end point, which adjusted for gender, age, statin use at randomization, duration from last MI, together with total and HDL-cholesterol produced a 13% reduction in risk (90.87, CI 0.76–0.99; p = 0.04). The secondary end point was major CVD events (coronary events plus stroke), which was the primary end point in TNT; this was significantly reduced by 13% (0.87, CI 0.78–0.98; p = 0.02). There was no difference in overall mortality or cancer deaths between the groups but the trial was not powered on overall mortality. There were more drug discontinuations in the atorvastatin group but given the PROBE design and the fact that 51% of patients recruited were already taking simvastatin there may be some reporting bias. Central laboratory results, however, were blinded and there were significantly more withdrawals due to elevated liver function in the atorvastatin group (1% vs 0.1%) (Pedersen et al. 2005).

The Pravastatin or Atorvastatin Evaluation and Infection Therapy: Thrombolysis in Myocardial Infarction 22 (PROVE-IT-TIMI 22) assessed standard compared to conventional statin therapy in patients with ACS (Cannon et al. 2004). This trial was designed as a non-inferiority trial of pravastatin compared to atorvastatin. A total of 4,162 ACS patients were randomized to pravastatin 40mg/day compared to atorvastatin 80mg/day within 10 days of the event. The primary end point was a composite of death, non-fatal MI, unstable angina requiring hospitalization, stroke, and revascularization, performed at least 30 days after randomization. In the pravastatin group, the mean LDL was 2.46mmol/L and in the atovastatin group 1.6mmol/L and this difference was associated with a 16% risk reduction (CI 5–26%; p = 0.005) in favour of the atorvastatin group after a mean 2-yr follow-up. Reduction in the rate of death was 28%, which was of borderline significance (p = 0.07). Of interest was the early separation of the event curves the benefit with the more intensive regimen being apparent at 30 days (Cannon *et al.* 2004).

A prespecified analysis of the diabetic patients included in the PROVE-IT trial has been reported (Ahmed *et al.* 2006). A total of 978 patients with diabetes were identified on the basis of clinical history, fasting glucose ≥126mg/dL (7mmol/L), or haemoglobin A1c >7% and compared to 3,184 patients without diabetes. The rate of acute cardiac events, death, myocardial infarction, and unstable angina requiring hospitalization was considerably higher in those with diabetes but was reduced by intensive treatment 21.1% versus 26.6% (HR=0.75, p = 0.03) compared to 14% versus 18% (HR=0.76, p = 0.002) in those without diabetes, p for interaction 0.97. In those with diabetes, 55 events were saved per 1,000 patients treated compared to 44 in those without diabetes.

A second trial has examined the impact of statin therapy in ACS patients. In phase Z of the A-Z trial (Aggrastat® to Zocor®), 4,497 patients were randomized to either simvastatin 40mg/day for 1 month then increasing to 80mg/day, or placebo for 4 months. At 4 months, those patients on placebo received 20mg/day and the trial continued for at least 6 months and up to 24 months (median follow-up, 721 days) (de Lemos *et al.* 2004). LDL was reduced from 2.88mmol/L to 2.1mmol/L in the low-dose group compared to 1.7mmol/L in the high-dose group. At 1 month on simvastatin 40mg/day LDL was 1.76mmol/L and at 4 months on simvastatin 80mg/day it was 1.6mmol/L. Despite these reductions, there was no benefit observed at 4 months and at the end of the study, the primary end point was not achieved. However, in a *post hoc* analysis, from 4 months through to the end of the study the primary end point was reduced from 9.3% in the placebo plus simvastatin group to 6.8% in the simvastatin only group (0.75, CI 0.6–0.95; p = 0.02). On simvastatin 80mg/day, there were nine patients with myopathy compared with none in the low-dose group and one in the placebo group. The authors commented that 'clinicians should be aware that the 80mg/day dose of simvastatin is associated with a higher risk of myopathy than lower dosages of the drug and should educate patients receiving the 80mg/day dose of simvastatin to pay close attention to muscle-related symptoms' (de Lemos *et al.* 2004).

Much has been written in an attempt to explain the different outcomes of A-Z and PROVE-IT. It may be that the explanation relates to the failure in A-Z to use high-dose statin in the first month. Certainly, there is a difference in C-reactive protein response with no change in this inflammatory marker in A-Z compared to significant reduction in PROVE-IT. Other possibilities may involve differences in recruitment time following ACS with more patients in A-Z less likely to undergo coronary intervention than in PROVE-IT. Nevertheless, it is only atorvastatin 80mg/day that has been shown to reduce early and late CVD events following ACS.

These four trials have been subjected to meta-analysis to gain further insight into the potential benefits of more intensive treatment. As the trials had some differences in their primary end points or definitions used, the meta-analysis adopted the following end points to compare the four trials: (1) combined incidence of coronary death or non-fatal MI; (2) combined incidence of coronary death or any CVD event; (3) the incidence of stroke; and (4) incidence of CVD, non-CVD, and all-cause mortality. In the pooled analysis, approximately one-quarter of patients were on statin at baseline and LDL fell by 22% to a mean of 2.59mmol/L on standard therapy and by 42% to 1.92mmol/L on intensive therapy, giving a mean difference of 25.7% between the two treatment groups. Pooled analysis of coronary death and non-fatal MI showed a significant reduction of 16% (0.84, CI 0.77–0.91; p < 0.00001) (see Figure 10.1). Stroke was reduced by 18% (0.82, CI 0.71–0.96; p = 0.012). There was a non-significant trend towards reduction in CVD death (0.88, 0.78–1.00; p = 0.054). There were no significant changes in non-CVD deaths or overall mortality. This comprehensive analysis, based on 100,000 patient-years of observation is a compelling point to the extra benefits of more intensive therapy in high-risk individuals. The authors calculated that for every million patients with chronic or acute coronary disease treated for 5yrs, there would be a saving of 35,000 CVD events and a number needed to treat of 29 over 2yrs for ACS and 5yrs for stable disease (Cannon et al. 2006).

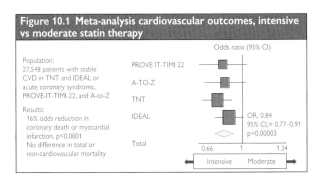

Figure 10.1 Meta-analysis cardiovascular outcomes, intensive vs moderate statin therapy

Population:
27,548 patients with stable CVD in TNT and IDEAL or acute coronary syndrome, PROVE-IT-TIMI-22, and A-to-Z

Results:
16% odds reduction in coronary death or myocardial infarction, p<0.0001
No difference in total or non-cardiovascular mortality

Odds ratio (95% CI)

PROVE IT-TIMI 22
A-TO-Z
TNT
IDEAL — OR, 0.84 95% CI,= 0.77–0.91 p=0.00003
Total

0.66   1   1.34

Intensive   Moderate

10.4 **What is the target LDL-cholesterol in high-risk patients?**

Given new information from RCTs, the National Cholesterol Education Program (NCEP) Adult Treatment Panel III in the United States produced an updated report to assess the impact of new RCT data for clinical management (Grundy *et al.* 2004). This report concluded that the new data confirmed the benefits of cholesterol-lowering for high-risk individuals and supported the target of <2.6mmol/L (100mg/dL). The new trials also supported treatment in people with diabetes and older people. In addition, they proposed a revised LDL target in those judged to be at very high risk of <1.8mmol/L (70mg/dL) as a therapeutic option.

Despite this considered view from NCEP and indeed from other consensus guideline groups such as the Joint British Societies in the United Kingdom (Joint British Societies 2005), there has been considerable debate concerning the lower LDL-cholesterol targets. In some health care systems, this relates to cost as the achievement of lower targets will necessitate the use of more potent statins not yet off patent and therefore more expensive. These political considerations apart, the clinician needs to balance the added benefit of more intensive therapy against a slight increase in adverse events. This does not seem to be an impediment in practice as the 1–2% incidence of raised (>3-fold) liver function tests with atorvastatin 80mg/day do not appear to be associated with clinical disease and revert to normal on reducing or stopping the drug. Patients should also be warned to stop the drugs in the event of severe muscle pain and tenderness to avoid myositis and possible rhabdomyolysis. The clinician needs to exercise due care in avoiding the potential for drug interactions, particularly drugs that inhibit CYP enzymes concerned with the metabolism of statins.

Some commentators have emphasized the fact that the new trials do not show benefit on overall mortality, failing to mention that the trials were not powered for this end point. In fact, because of improvements in cardiac care and secondary prevention, mortality rates are much lower now than when the 4S study was performed, which was powered on overall mortality (The Scandinavian Simvastatin Survival Study Group 1994). In 4S, CVD mortality was between 9% and 10% in the placebo group and non-cardiac mortality was about 2%, whereas in recent trials non-cardiac mortality at 3–5% is higher than CVD mortality at 2–3%. Commentators have pointed to slight non-significant increase in non-CVD mortality, which given the above discussion are likely to be the play of chance rather than drug-related and this is borne out by the meta-analysis (Cannon *et al.* 2006).

10.5 **Statins and stroke prevention**

As discussed in this chapter, an important bonus observed in the statin trials was the reduction in stroke (Amarenco et al. 2004). However, it is important to note that this observation related to the primary prevention of stroke in patients with established coronary disease or at moderate to high risk of CVD. Only limited data were available for the prevention of recurrent stroke in patients with previous stroke. For instance in HPS, no reduction was observed in the risk of stroke in patients with prior CVD treated with simvastatin 40mg/day (Heart Protection Study Collaborative Group 2002).

The first specific trial of the secondary prevention of stroke is the Stroke Prevention by Aggressive Reduction in Cholesterol Levels (SPARCL) trial (SPARCL Investigators 2006). SPARCL included 4,731 patients with previous stroke or transient ischaemic attack (TIA) within 1–6 months prior to study entry but no known coronary disease and LDL levels, 2.9–4.9mmol/L. Patients were randomized to receive atorvastatin 80mg/day or placebo and the primary end point was first fatal or non-fatal stroke. After a median follow-up of 4.9yrs, there was a 16% (0.84, 95% CI 0.71–0.99; p = 0.03) reduction in the primary end point, an absolute reduction in risk of 2.2%. Major CVD events were reduced by 20% (0.80, 0.69–0.92; p = 0.002). There was no difference in overall mortality. The net difference in statin use was 78% because of drop-in therapy in the placebo group and discontinuation in the active group. This is reflected in the LDL differences between the groups which was 53% at 1 month (1.58 vs 3.45mmol/L) but this became less over the course of the study (1.89 vs 3.32mmol/L). In a *post hoc* analysis, it was shown that the reduction in the primary end point was due to a 22% reduction in ischaemic stroke and there was a small but significant increase in haemorrhagic stroke. Of the 88 patients who had at least one haemorrhagic stroke, 55 were in the atorvastatin group and 33 in the placebo group. There was no difference in fatal haemorrhagic events (Amarenco et al. 2004). Of interest, there was a non-significant increase in haemorrhagic stroke (21 vs 11) in patients with prior cerebrovascular disease in HPS (Heart Protection Study Collaborative Group 2002) and epidemiologic associations have been described between low LDL-cholesterol and haemorrhagic stroke (Yano et al. 1989). Importantly, no increase in haemorrhagic stroke has been observed in other trials which have reduced LDL-cholesterol to approximately 1.8mmol/L.

Recently, the findings of SPARCL have been analysed in detail in relation to haemorrhagic stroke (Goldstein et al. 2007). Multiple regression analysis showed that the risk of haemorrhagic stroke was increased in those who entered the study with a baseline haemorrhagic stroke (HR 5.65, CI 2.82–11.30; p < 0.001), in men (HR

1.79, CI 1.13–2.84; p = 0.01), and with increasing age (10yr increments, HR 1.42, CI 1.16–1.74; p = 0.001). In addition, hypertension (systolic >160mmHg or diastolic >100mmHg) at the last visit prior to a haemorrhagic event, predicted risk, but there was no relationship between baseline or on-treatment LDL. In addition, atorvastatin treatment was related to increased risk (HR 1.68, CI 1.09–2.59; p = 0.02). These factors, other than treatment allocation, accounted for 86% of the increased risk of haemorrhagic events. However, they explain only a tiny proportion of the overall risk (about 1%). The authors concluded that 'in making therapeutic decisions, the increase in the risk of haemorrhagic stroke found in SPARCL, if not due to chance, must be balanced against the benefit of treatment with atorvastatin 80mg/day in reducing the overall risk of stroke, as well as other cardiovascular events found in the study's pre-specified, intention-to-treat analysis' (Goldstein et al. 2007).

References

Ahmed S, Cannon CP, Murphy SA, and Braunwald E (2006). Acute coronary syndromes and diabetes: is intensive lipid lowering beneficial? Results of the PROVE IT-TIMI 22 trial. *European Heart Journal*, **27**, 2323–9.

Amarenco P, Labreuche J, Lavallee P, et al. (2004) Statins in stroke prevention and carotid atherosclerosis: systematic review and meta-analysis. *Stroke*, **35**, 2902–9.

Cannon CP, Braunwald E, McCabe CH, et al. (2004). Intensive versus moderate lipid lowering with statins after coronary syndromes. *The New England Journal of Medicine*, **350**, 1495–504.

Cannon CP, Steinberg BA, Murphy SA, et al. (2006). Meta-analysis of cardiovascular outcomes trials comparing intensive versus moderate statin therapy. *Journal of the American College of Cardiology*, **48**, 438–45.

Cholesterol Treatment Trialists' (CTT) Collaboration (2005). Efficacy and safety of cholesterol-lowering treatment: prospective meta-analysis of data from 90,056 participants in 14 randomised trials. *The Lancet*, **366**, 1267–78.

de Lemos JA, Blazing MA, Wiviott SD, et al. (2004). Early intensive vs delayed conservative simvastatin strategy in patients with acute coronary syndromes. Phase Z of the A to Z Trial. *JAMA*, **292**, 1307–16.

Goldstein LB, Amarenco P, Szarek M, et al. (2007). Secondary analysis of haemorrhagic stroke in the Stroke Prevention by Aggressive Reduction in Cholesterol Levels (SPARCL) Study. *Neurology*, **70**, 2364–70.

Grundy SM, Cleeman JI, Merz CNB, et al. (2004). Implications of recent clinical trials for the National Cholesterol Education Program Adult Treatment Panel III Guidelines. *Circulation*, **110**, 227–39.

Heart Protection Study Collaborative Group (2002). MRC/BHF Heart Protection Study of cholesterol lowering with simvastatin in 20,536 high risk individuals: a randomized placebo-controlled trial. *The Lancet*, **360**, 7–22.

Joint British Societies (2005). Guidelines for prevention of cardiovascular disease in clinical practice. JBS 2. *Heart*, **91**(Suppl V), v1–52.

LaRosa JC, Grundy SM, Waters DD, *et al.* (2005). Intensive lipid lowering with atorvastatin in patients with stable coronary disease. *The New England Journal of Medicine*, **352**, 1425–35.

Pedersen TR, Faergeman O, Kastelein JJP, *et al.* (2005). High-dose atorvastatin vs usual-dose simvastatin for secondary prevention after myocardial infarction. The IDEAL Study: a randomized controlled trial. *JAMA*, **294**, 2437–45.

Shepherd J, Barter P, Carmena R, *et al.* (2006) Effect of lowering LDL cholesterol substantially below recommended levels in patients with coronary heart disease: the Treating to New Targets (TNT) Study. *Diabetes Care*, **29**, 1220–6.

The Scandinavian Simvastatin Survival Study Group (1994). Randomised trial of cholesterol lowering in 4444 people with coronary heart disease: the Scandinavian simvastatin survival study (4S). *The Lancet*, **344**,1383–9.

The Stroke Prevention by Aggressive Reduction in Cholesterol Levels (SPARCL) Investigators (2006). High dose atorvastatin after stroke or transient ischaemic attack. *The New England Journal of Medicine*, **355**, 549–59.

Yano K, Reed DM, and MacLean CJ. (1989) Serum cholesterol and haemorrhagic stroke in the Honolulu Heart programme. *Stroke*, **20**, 1460–5.

Chapter 11

Vascular imaging

Manish Kalla and Julian Halcox

Key points

- Atherosclerosis is a dynamic process that affects most medium and large calibre arteries, particularly the coronary and carotid arteries.
- Atherosclerotic changes in the arteries develop over many decades before clinical presentation.
- First cardiac events are often either myocardial infarction or death, with most acute coronary events triggered by destabilization and rupture of lipid, rich, thin capped, usually only mildly obstructive plaques.
- Early identification of subclinical atherosclerosis and high-risk plaque/preclinical disease is of value in assessing a patient's future risk of developing clinical disease.
- Angiography remains the gold standard investigation but visualizes only stenoses, which are a late manifestation of the atherosclerotic process.
- Newer modalities such as computed tomography (CT) angiography, B mode carotid ultrasound, and magnetic resonance imaging (MRI) can identify at-risk individuals without invasive investigations.
- Functional and anatomical imaging together holds great promise in for accurate identification of patients with high-risk plaque.

11.1 Introduction

This chapter will focus on established and emerging technologies in imaging the coronary and carotid vascular systems. Disease in these territories often presents acutely leading to significant morbidity and mortality. Thus, our review aims to define optimal methods for assessing burden and risk of atherosclerotic disease, recognizing that emerging modalities have the potential to identify plaque pathophysiology and risk of acute destabilization. This will not only allow identification and stratification of vascular risk, but also help guide selection and development of preventive therapies. Arterial imaging has progressed rapidly over recent years. In the field of cardiology, coronary angiography remains the gold standard, and greater progress has been made in terms of diagnosis and clinical research end points, and in the use of emerging imaging technology for identification and characterization of the pathophysiological process of atherosclerosis in the vessel wall. Evaluation of the effect of risk factor modification through lifestyle and pharmacological interventions has also benefited from the use of non-invasive imaging to detect disease progression or regression, as well as improving our ability to select high-risk patients that may derive most benefit from invasive management. Furthermore, the intensive effort to develop newer modalities for more safe and accurate identification of preclinical disease has been driven by the observation that atherosclerotic disease more often than not presents catastrophically, with over 50% of patients who develop atherosclerosis in their lifetime presenting with death or a myocardial infarction as their first event.

11.2 **Pathophysiology**

Atherosclerosis is a dynamic process affecting medium and large arteries. The disease is characterized by endothelial dysfunction, inflammation and deposition of lipid, cellular components, and calcium within the intimal layer. The end product of this multifactorial process is a plaque which may increase in size resulting in vessel stenosis, reduction in blood flow leading to symptoms of end organ ischaemia, and importantly, the plaque may also rupture leading to acute thrombosis and damage to the tissue subtended downstream of the occlusion.

Pathophysiological mechanisms leading to the development of atherosclerotic plaque include endothelial injury by factors such as oxidative and shear stresses, which promote endothelial dysfunction platelet adhesion, lipid uptake, and smooth muscle proliferation.

The earliest manifestation of these processes is the fatty streak, which progresses to form a fibrous plaque by ongoing lipid accumulation and migration and proliferation of smooth muscle cells. Plaque growth leads to positive remodelling with preservation of lumen diameter, but eventually luminal narrowing occurs. This increase in size is associated with neovascularization within the plaque which increases the risk of haemorrhage and plaque rupture. Ongoing endothelial damage and denudation or rupture of the fibrous plaque exposes the thrombogenic core of lipids, resulting in a cascade of cytokine activation and cellular aggregation leading to acute coronary syndromes or cerebrovascular events. Imaging techniques that are able to identify and measure plaque are currently available, and biological techniques to image the key cellular and metabolic processes involved in plaque progression and destabilization are in active development.

11.3 Coronary angiography and intravascular ultrasound (IVUS)

Coronary angiography, introduced in 1959 by Mason Sones and colleagues, remains the gold standard modality for assessing coronary disease. This technique involves imaging the outline of the arterial lumen in multiple planes by direct intracoronary injection of radio-opaque contrast medium. This identifies stenotic disease and also allows therapeutic intervention to be delivered if needed. Many landmark trials have utilized angiography to define the relationship between risk factors and coronary stenoses with many early trials demonstrating worsening prognosis in relation to increasing number of coronary vessels with obstructive stenoses.

Advantages of coronary angiography
- Widely available
- Reliable, reproducible, and validated
- Diagnostic and therapeutic (if indicated).

Limitations of coronary angiography
- Invasive procedure with 0.1–1% risk of major complications including vascular damage, contrast nephropathy, stroke, myocardial infarction, and death
- Only visualizes lumen stenosis, which is usually a late feature of atherosclerosis
- Underestimates disease severity when compared with pathological samples.

11.4 Intravascular ultrasound

One major disadvantage of angiography is that it only demonstrates changes in the calibre and contour of the lumen. Early disease development typically progresses eccentrically with expansive plaque growth into the vessel wall rather than into the lumen (positive remodelling). Thus, significant plaque volume may accumulate, including unstable plaque, without evidence of significant stenosis, or limitation of blood flow as defined angiographically.

This limitation has been addressed by intravascular ultrasound (IVUS), which allows quantification of not only luminal area but also plaque volume along the length of an artery. It is also an invasive technique that involves passing a catheter with an ultrasound transducer at the tip along a guidewire into a coronary artery, and withdrawing it at a constant speed resulting in a cross-sectional image being displayed on a monitor. This technique was first introduced as an aid to percutaneous intervention, but experience has defined its role in assessing plaque composition and remodelling including identification of vulnerable or ruptured plaque (Figure 11.1). Although its use has been limited to high risk or symptomatic patients who are already undergoing invasive investigation, IVUS has shown that disease progression can be constrictive leading to a reduction in lumen area or stenosis as visualized by conventional angiography or expansive (positive) without causing flow limitation. IVUS has been used in research trials addressing effective stent delivery and has been able to quantify accurately changes in plaque volume following pharmacological risk factor modification; for example, regression of atheroma with high potency statin therapy (Table 11.1).

Owing to its invasive nature, coronary angiography with or without IVUS is only appropriate for use in the management of those patients who have already developed symptoms of cardiac ischaemia (Table 11.2). It is, therefore, not appropriate for identifying patients during the long preclinical phase of disease, as the risk–benefit ratio of using an invasive method with significant (albeit infrequent) complications does not support its use as a screening tool. Therefore, many other modalities have been developed that are more appropriate for wider use in identifying the various manifestations of atherosclerotic disease.

11.5 CT: coronary artery calcification (CAC) and angiography

Vascular calcification occurs almost exceptionally in the setting of atherosclerosis. Calcium deposition is an active process resulting from chronic inflammation, which leads to the expression of bone structural proteins and calcium phosphate crystal uptake by macrophages within plaques. Furthermore, plaque development is aided by neovascularization and associations have been observed between new vessel formation and calcification. Furthermore, calcified lesions on IVUS tend to signify stable stenotic lesions, and in this setting usually represent a late manifestation of atherosclerosis.

Calcium deposited within plaque can be identified utilizing various computed tomography (CT) modalities, including electron beam CT (EBCT), conventional helical CT (HCT), and more recently multiple row multidetector CT (MDCT). This can be quantified and presented as a coronary artery calcium score (Agaston score), which is a validated indicator of chronic plaque burden.

Figure 11.1 Coronary angiography with additional insights gained from IVUS

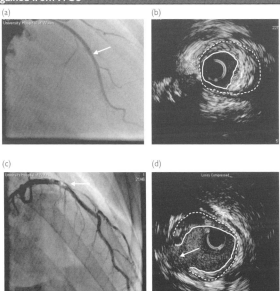

(a)   (b)

(c)   (d)

Panels (a) and (b) show an angiogram of the left anterior descending artery (a) with some minor irregularities in the mid segment (arrow) and the IVUS appearances (b) at the point identified by the arrow in (a). Significant atheroma is observed in the subintimal area (region bounded by the continuous and dashed lines). There is significant positive remodelling in the vessel producing an unobstructed luminal appearance on the angiogram. Panels (c) and (d) show an angiogram (c) demonstrating an area of severe disease in the proximal left anterior descending artery (arrow) with the IVUS image in the corresponding region (d) demonstrating plaque with evidence of rupture (arrow).

Table 11.1 Role of IVUS

Risk stratification of plaque	Clinical applications
• Ultrasound can identify calcification • Constrictive plaques show extensive calcification • Expansive plaques are less calcified and more fibro-fatty • Expansive morphology is associated with plaque instability • Most non-fatal coronary events occur due to rupture and thrombotic occlusion of mildly obstructive plaque	• Assessment of moderate lesions on angiography • Left main disease • High-risk plaque • Coronary dissection • Optimizing stent delivery • Follow up in cardiac transplant patients

Table 11.2 Coronary angiography and IVUS
• Widely available, reliable, and validated techniques
• IVUS improves on limitations of angiography by visualizing lumen and wall pathologies
• IVUS can identify high-risk plaques
• Invasive nature makes them unsuitable for screening at-risk groups

Despite not identifying high-risk lipid-rich plaques, higher CAC scores indirectly reflect an increased likelihood of high-risk plaque similar to those with the greatest disease burden are more likely to have one or more such lesions. Thus, the CAC score also predicts increased risk of cardiac events, with recent meta-analyses demonstrating a roughly twofold increase in relative risk for Agaston scores between 1 and 100 and adjusted relative risks ranging between 3 and 17 for higher calcium scores. Its clinical role has been considered by the ACC and the AHA, who felt it is appropriate for use in further evaluation of cardiovascular risk in asymptomatic patients concerned about their cardiovascular risk. Greatest incremental predictive value of CAC imaging was felt to be in patients found to be at intermediate cardiovascular risk (10–20% 10-year risk of MI or stroke) by conventional risk factor assessment methods, with more aggressive investigation and treatment recommended for those found to have higher CAC scores.

Over the past few years, MDCT angiography (MDCTA) use has increased as technological advances allow faster acquisition of images of epicardial arteries and CAC with increasing detail (Figure 11.2). Studies typically require 80–100mL of iodinated contrast and only take a few minutes to perform. Numerous studies have validated MDCTA against coronary angiography in determining luminal obstruction, with results showing >90% sensitivity, specificity, positive and negative predictive to the detection of major epicardial vessel stenosis of >50% severity in patients without previously known atherosclerosis. Accuracy may be affected by the presence of stents, fast or irregular heart rates, and extensive vascular calcification. Its main application in clinical practice centres on its high negative predictive value and ability to exclude significant coronary stenosis in patients with low to intermediate risk in whom an angiographic diagnosis is felt to be of clinical value. In addition, it is of use in low-intermediate risk patients with equivocal or suspected false positive stress testing, thereby avoiding invasive angiography. Drawbacks include higher effective radiation dose compared with diagnostic angiography, artefact due to stents or calcification, overestimation of stenoses with no information on the functional significance of lesions. Improving technology is expected to diminish these latter concerns in the next few years (Table 11.3).

Figure 11.2 CT coronary angiography (MDCT)

(a)   (b)

(c)   (d)

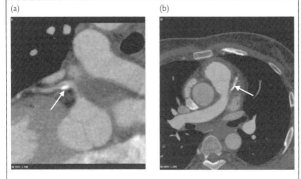

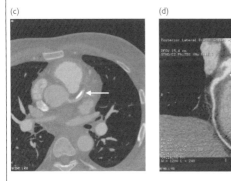

CT coronary angiography (MDCT) showing plaque with heterogeneous composition (arrow), including calcification, in the proximal left anterior descending artery (panels a–c). (d) shows an aneurysmal proximal segment of the right coronary artery with a filling defect suggestive of thrombus (arrow).

Table 11.3 Key points: CT for CAC and CTA

- Widely available, automated, and reliable modality
- CAC identifies disease burden and predicts coronary events
- CTA provides reliable and validated assessment of stenosis in epicardial coronary arteries with high negative predictive value
- Limited by artefact from stents or heavy calcification
- MDCTA most useful for lumen/plaque assessment populations with low-intermediate pretest probability of obstructive disease in whom an angiographic diagnosis is required

11.6 **Cardiac magnetic resonance imaging (CMR)**

CMR does not expose the patient to radiation and does not require potentially nephrotoxic intravenous contrast, although concerns have been recently raised regarding potential nephrotoxicity of gadolinium MR contrast agents. Despite rapid advances in coronary magnetic resonance imaging (MRI), it currently has lower sensitivity and specificity than MDCT for vascular imaging. Scanning takes 40min and accuracy can be limited by lower spatial resolution than CT.

At present, CMR is used clinically for the assessment of heart and great vessel morphology as well as cardiac function and viability, without the acoustic window limitations of echocardiography.

Current CMR research is evaluating combined coronary artery imaging with the assessment of myocardial perfusion and regional wall motion abnormalities, which could improve the diagnostic ease and accuracy of functional and structural computer-aided design (CAD). Furthermore, there should be less potential to generate false-negative results than with nuclear perfusion imaging where a global reduction in blood flow with balanced defects may sometimes appear to uniformly normal perfusion with stress.

Progress in arterial imaging has not been confined to the coronary system. Imaging carotid atherosclerosis is key due to its relationship with cerebrovascular events and also its correlation with coronary atherosclerosis, particularly the extent of disease in the wall of the coronary vessels. Thus, imaging of the carotid arteries has also provided further insight into the biology of plaque development.

MRI is ideally suited to define atherosclerosis. Images obtained can detail lumen size, wall architecture, and also provide valuable information on plaque composition including cap thickness and integrity (rupture), calcification, lipid core, and neovasculature. Thus, remodelling can also be assessed with sequential MRI, and early data have shown plaque regression and reduction in lipid core with statin therapy. *In vivo* wall and plaque characteristics by MRI are closely correlated to histopathological features of specimens subsequently removed at carotid endarterectomy. Furthermore, high-risk plaque characteristics defined by MRI (thin or ruptured fibrous cap, intraplaque haemorrhage, increased lipid core volume, and increased wall thickness) have been shown to be associated with increased incidence of cerebrovascular events (hazard ratios 1.6–17). However, these data are from small studies and larger prospective studies will be required to provide further confirmation of these associations and allow assessment of potential clinical utility.

Advantages of MRI include its non-invasive approach and assessment of all components of the atherosclerotic process. Drawbacks to its integration into routine clinical practice include its expense and time (imaging time is approximately 45min), lower availability, and limited spatial resolution. These issues, particularly temporospatial resolution have also limited its utilization for assessing coronary arteries. Nevertheless, MRI has great promise in increasing understanding of atherosclerosis, while longer-term studies will define its role in identifying a clinical role for characterization of and management guidance in higher-risk patients.

11.7 **B-mode ultrasound**

Early experience with ultrasound in the 1970s utilized Doppler signalling to measure flow within carotid arteries. These data were then quantified to determine a percentage stenosis of the artery lumen. By focusing on luminal stenosis rather than the atherogenic processes in the arterial wall, clinical use of this modality remained limited to the assessment of subjects with more advanced obstructive disease.

The development of B-mode ultrasound addressed this limitation by allowing accurate imaging of arterial walls. Further advantages included relative ease of use, portability, reproducibility, good axial resolution, and semiautomated identification between lumen and layers of the arterial wall and lesion characteristics (Figure 11.3). These advantages have made its use central to many large multicentre epidemiological studies and clinical trials that have increased understanding of the pathogenesis and natural history of atherosclerosis.

Figure 11.3 **Carotid B-mode ultrasound and IMT detection**

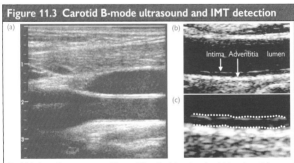

Panel (a) shows the common carotid artery bifurcating into external and internal carotid arteries. Panel (b) demonstrates the detection of common carotid arterial lumen, intima, and adventitia (distal bright line). The IMT is bounded by the lumen-intima and adventitial interfaces and comprises the intima, subintimal, and media. Panel (c) shows an enlarged image of the far wall of the arterial segment shown in (b), illustrating the use of edge detection software. This can be used to calculate a mean IMT and also define the maximal IMT within a user-defined region of interest in the vessel.

Wall thickness and, especially, the component of the wall delineated between the lumen-intima and media-adventitia interfaces, better known as the carotid IMT (intimal-medial thickness). IMT is the measurement used by most investigators to define early arterial pathophysiology, which probably reflects both fibromuscular hyperplasia and atheroma of the vessel wall. Whilst it is difficult to distinguish between the different pathophysiological components, most investigators believe that the extent of the increase in wall thickness is an adequate marker of advancing vascular disease. Increased IMT is associated with expansive remodelling of the common carotid artery and most CAD risk factors are associated with increasing IMT. Whilst intima-medial thickening is generally a diffuse process, plaque formation that typically affects the region of the carotid bulb and bifurcation where focal initiation and progression of disease is promoted by disrupted shear forces affecting the vascular endothelium.

As with MRI, carotid IMT and plaque correlate well with changes in the coronary arteries, particularly changes in the wall characterized by IVUS. Current data suggest that IMT can be used as a surrogate marker for coronary atherosclerosis and to identify individuals at increased future cardiovascular risk (IMT ≥1mm, IMT ≥75th age and gender predicted centile, or the presence of carotid plaque).

Contrast-enhanced ultrasound of the carotid system has provided further insight into identifying high-risk plaque and patients. Localized ischaemia leads to the release of angiogenic factors by promoting new vessel formation within plaque. This process is typically more exuberant in plaque that is more metabolically active, and rich in lipid and inflammatory cells. These are typically features of vulnerable plaque and intraplaque haemorrhage from this neovasculature is a further recognized mechanism associated with plaque rupture and occlusive events. Intravenous contrast highlights tissue planes for identifying IMT and lesions not seen with two-dimensional imaging, while intraplaque contrast enhancement identifies neovascularization and therefore high-risk plaque. Quantification of this potentially important process requires validation and standardization.

11.8 **IMT and coronary artery disease**

- CAD patients have greater IMT and more rapid IMT progression than patients with CVD risk factors
- Increased IMT and/or presence of carotid plaque predicts an increased risk myocardial infarction and stroke
- IMT is significantly correlated with post-mortem coronary atheroma and IVUS-defined coronary atheroma, but less consistently correlated with coronary luminal stenosis by quantitative coronary angiography.

Table 11.4 Key points: B mode carotid ultrasound and IMT

- Widely available, portable, and reproducible
- Assessment of two key arterial systems (indirect inference of coronary pathology)
- Images all aspects of atherosclerotic process
- Non-invasive prediction of risk of coronary and cerebrovascular events
- Modest improvement on conventional risk stratification scores, e.g. Framingham, most informative in intermediate risk individuals
- Less accurate than CT CAC at identifying patients with 'angiographically stenotic' CAD, but similar prediction of adverse cardiovascular outcome

- IMT has been used in many clinical trials to demonstrate the efficacy of pharmacological interventions on preclinical disease. Statin therapy has consistently shown either slowing of progression or regression of IMT, antihypertensive therapy slows progression, and intensive control of glycaemia in diabetes show similar but less predictable effects on IMT (Table 11.4).

11.9 Endothelial function testing

Endothelial dysfunction is the earliest fundamental component of atherogenesis, which continues throughout the evolution of the disease. Investigators have developed non-invasive techniques to identify individuals with endothelial dysfunction that reflect risk factor exposure, correlate with impaired coronary reactivity, and have been shown to predict subsequent adverse cardiac events and are only just being considered for use as clinical tests. It is unlikely that evaluation of endothelial function will be widely used outside of the research setting, but some subgroups of challenging patients may benefit including those with ischaemic-type chest pain and unobstructed coronary arteries.

11.10 FMD and coronary events

- Attenuated flow-mediated dilation (FMD) is predictive of long-term cardiovascular events in patients with atherosclerosis
- Recent data have shown similar correlation with reactive hyperaemia
- Framingham study has suggested a stronger correlation between cardiovascular risk factors and reactive hyperaemia, and researchers speculate this may reflect microvascular dysfunction as part of early atherogenesis
- FMD alterations may represent established cardiovascular disease
- FMD unlikely to be part of mainstream vascular assessment.

11.11 **The future**

Most of the modalities reviewed primarily define coronary or carotid lumen loss, with B-mode IMT, IVUS CMR able to provide additional information on plaque composition. The ideal investigation would obtain data characterizing not only lumen change and arterial wall characteristics but also information regarding the biological activity of the vascular wall and plaque when present. Studies have shown that high-risk, rupture prone plaques are characterized by increased inflammatory cells and proteins. This feature can be targeted by positron emission tomography (PET), which utilizes fluorine-18 labelled deoxyglucose uptake by metabolically active cells to identify these plaques. Combined with the ability of CT to define CAC, wall thickening, and luminal changes, PET-CT may be the future tool of choice in identifying at-risk populations, albeit limited by radiation dose. Novel PET tracers bound to biological ligands are likely to provide unprecedented insights into the *in vivo* pathophysiology of atherosclerosis. To date, this modality remains the focus of intensive ongoing research efforts. Some potential limitations include small plaque size, cardiac motion artefact, and myocardial uptake of tracer.

11.12 **Conclusions**

Arterial imaging has developed rapidly since the first analyses of pathological samples. The ideal modality that not only images all aspects of the atherosclerotic process; walls, lumen, and plaque activity remains the holy grail, but also combinations of investigations may provide a holistic appraisal of an individual cardiovascular risk. Coronary angiography will not be replaced in the acute coronary syndrome setting as percutaneous interventional therapy is often required. However, defining the location and burden of disease and refinement of prognostication is well served by non-invasive modalities such as coronary CT and carotid ultrasound in low-intermediate risk groups. In the future, biological imaging with PET-CT and nanotechnology are likely to provide key insights into the disease and may command an important role in cardiovascular risk assessment of and selection of and measurement of the response to preventive therapies.

Acknowledgements

The authors are grateful to Dr. Tim Kinnaird, Dr. Andrew Wood, and Ms. Libby Ellins (University Hospital of Wales and Cardiff University) for kindly providing images included in this chapter.

References

Amato M, Montorsi P, Ravani A, *et al.* (2007). Carotid intima-media thickness by B-mode ultrasound as surrogate of coronary atherosclerosis: correlation with quantitative coronary angiography and coronary intravascular ultrasound findings. *European Heart Journal*, **28**, 2094–101.

Crouse JR (2006). Imaging atherosclerosis: state of the art. *Journal of Lipid Research*, **47**, 1677–99.

Feinstein SB (2006). Contrast ultrasound imaging of the carotid artery vasa vasorum and atherosclerotic plaque neovascularisation. *Journal of the American College of Cardiology*, **48**, 236–43.

Greenland P, Abrams J, Aurigemma GP, *et al.* (2000). Writing Group III. Prevention Conference V. Beyond Secondary Prevention: identifying the high-risk patient for primary prevention. Non-invasive tests of atherosclerotic burden. *Circulation*, **101**, E16–22.

Moens AL, Goovaerts I, Claeys MJ, *et al.* (2005). Flow-mediated vasodilatation: a diagnostic instrument, or an experimental tool. *Chest*, **127**, 2254–63.

Pletcher MJ, Tice JA, Pigone M, *et al.* (2004). Using the coronary artery calcium score to predict coronary heart disease events: a systematic review and meta-analysis. *Archives in Internal Medicine*, **164**, 1285–92.

Sanz J and Fayad ZA (2008). Imaging of atherosclerotic cardiovascular disease. *Nature*, **451**, 953–7.

Schwaiger M, Ziegler S, and Nekolla SG (2005). PET/CT: challenge for nuclear cardiology. *Journal of Nuclear Medicine*, **46**, 1664–1678.

Chapter 12

Common problems in lipid management

John Reckless

Key points

- Cholesterol and low-density lipoprotein (LDL)-cholesterol are causal factors for atheromatous cardiovascular disease (CVD), and moderate and higher levels are a near obligate for disease development.
- Statin drugs have overwhelming evidence of benefit at low side effect risk.
- Estimation of an individual's CVD risk is required from a number of factors, and CVD prevention requires attention to all abnormal modifiable factors in individuals at higher risk.
- Identifying, counselling, and appropriate treatment of individuals at high CVD risk is a current challenge for health care professionals.
- Guidelines have been produced to help, and Government has provided levers to encourage their application.

12.1 Background

Lipids and dyslipidaemia are important for the clinician in relation to their potential sequelae for the patient, primarily because of their role in risk for macrovascular disease—coronary, cerebral, and peripheral vascular disease. In addition, severe hypertriglyceridaemia can be associated with acute pancreatitis.

The causal relationship between low-density lipoprotein-cholesterol (LDL-C) and coronary heart disease (CHD) is clearly established, as is the inverse relationship between high-density lipoprotein-cholesterol (HDL-C) and CHD. Relative risk reduction by LDL-C lowering in randomized clinical trials (RCTs) is seen equally in different groups, in males and females, at ages up to 85yrs, with and without diabetes, in hypertension, and with other drug therapies. There currently does not seem to be a particular low level of LDL-C below which benefit ceases. Importantly, and despite the much flatter epidemiological relationship between cholesterol and stroke, LDL-C lowering with statins substantially reduces thrombotic stroke.

12.2 **Who should have treatment?—those at sufficient risk**

Cardiovascular disease (CVD) risk reflects multiple risk factors, main ones being sex, age, smoking, hypertension, total (specifically LDL) cholesterol, HDL-C, and diabetes, some being inevitable and some modifiable. It is an individual's total or global risk that needs addressing, and not an isolated factor. This may be in individuals already with overt clinical vascular disease in whom recurrence risk is high, but also individuals yet to manifest disease. Significant asymptomatic atheroma was demonstrated in young adults dying in war or road traffic accidents.

12.3 **Practical approaches to patients in the clinic**

Individuals attend their primary care team for various reasons providing opportunity for CVD assessment and management, but requiring organized approaches to identify individuals at high CVD risk. Some will already have CVD; others will have known risk factors while others will have none yet known. The primary care team should counsel individuals about CVD risk and assessment, why it may be important for them, and encourage acquisition of the key clinical data. After formal assessment, patients at significant risk need management to minimize that risk. In secondary care, a similar consideration should be made of a patient's CVD risk.

12.4 **The health care professional's problems in lipid management**

Has the individual patient got significant CVD risk? Why, and what (if anything) should be done? How is an individual's requirements integrated with those of the practice population?

An individual's lipid abnormalities need identifying with cholesterol/HDL-C ratio used with other factors to approximately quantify absolute CVD risk. A fasting sample will be needed for triglyceride and a calculated LDL-C. Thereafter, is intervention for lipids (and other risk factors) required?

Over two decades, the first target of lipid management has become LDL-C lowering with a statin in patients at sufficient risk. RCTs (Scandinavian Simvastatin Survival Study Group 1994; Heart Protection Study Collaborative Group 2002; Colhoun *et al.* 2004; Sever *et al.* 2004; Cholesterol Treatment Trialists' Collaborators 2005) have shown greater benefit of more intensive LDL-lowering over standard lowering, and from lower LDL baseline values, at least in secondary prevention. It is not established as to whether it should be percentage or absolute LDL-lowering or whether one should treat to 'a target'. Surrogate studies assessing changes in carotid intima-medial thickness (cIMT) or in coronary intravascular ultrasound (IVUS) have supported possible thresholds for LDL-C around 1.7mmol/L below which some regression of atheromatous plaques may occur. Achieving these LDL levels may require maximum doses (with somewhat higher adverse event rates) of combination therapy, but will not be possible with a single (statin) agent in all patients. Health care purchasers may not wish to meet the increased costs of using more potent (and non-generic) statins (National Institute for Health and Clinical Excellence 2007a; NICE GDG) or the addition of non-statin additional agents [such as NICE TA ezetimibe (National Institute for Health and Clinical Excellence 2007b)], which do not have long-term hard outcome data. Health economists may not consider the ICERs (incremental cost-effectiveness ratios) to be sufficiently good to warrant intensification of treatment. Within a fixed resource, there will be greater population benefits from using less costly generic agents in higher proportions of the target population than more expensive therapies in smaller numbers.

12.5 Making the diagnosis and initiating therapy

Measurement of a random cholesterol and HDL-C with other risk factors allows approximation of a patient's absolute CVD risk over 10yrs to be calculated using algorithms derived from the Framingham study (Anderson *et al.* 1991) (or other suitable risk calculation algorithms). These can be from charts such as those in the Joint British Societies' second guidelines (The Joint British Societies 2005), or from computer-based algorithms as standalone programs or embedded within primary care patient data management systems.

Drug treatment should not be initiated for primary prevention on a single measurement, and one measurement should be fasting including triglycerides to allow a calculated LDL-C. As first-line drug management (after lifestyle and dietary advice) will be a statin, LDL-C is a more specific target than total cholesterol. Secondary causes of a dyslipidaemia should be sought with liver, renal and thyroid function, glucose, obesity, and alcohol to be considered.

For secondary prevention, a statin will normally be initiated with other indicated treatments at the time of the acute event. Fasting lipid profiles and consideration of secondary disorder contributors should be revisited at 2–3 months follow up.

12.6 **Who are these at-risk groups who should be considered for treatment?**

Three main groups need consideration. First, those with clinical CVD in any territory have such high risk of further events that they should receive 'secondary' prevention treatment. Second, risks in diabetes (Cholesterol Treatment Trialists' Collaborators 2008) are 3- to 4-fold greater than without diabetes so all require assessment, and most will require management. The third and largest group is of individuals where combination of factors gives high risk, usually accepted as ≥20% chance of an event over 10yrs.

Within this third group are individuals with inherited lipid abnormalities evoking very high CVD risk. Familial hypercholesterolaemia (FH) affects 1 in 500 of the population. Untreated, half of males will have their first event by age 50 and around half will have died by age 60, with females being affected around 10yrs later. They need lifestyle and drug treatment from young adulthood, and it is mandatory for the clinician to identify affected first degree relatives. Cardiovascular risk has reduced with statin therapy, and likely lifestyle change has reduced cancer mortality in FH patients (Scientific Steering Committee on behalf of the Simon Broome Register Group 1999; Marks et al. 2003).

As all people have some risk, increasing with age, attention to lifestyle factors, avoidance of tobacco use, and fitness are relevant to all. However, pharmacotherapy should be considered in relation to absolute CVD risk, overall benefit (relative risk reduction) of treatment, and risks of therapy. The benefit/risk ratio will vary for different treatments for lipids, blood pressure, or diabetes. Persist hypertension (>160/100mmHg), hypertension with target organ damage, cholesterol/HDL-C ratio ≥7.0, or familial dyslipidaemia are all indications to consider single factor treatment even when risk is estimated as <20%/10yr.

Even when CVD risk is as low as ≤10%/10yr for some treatments, there is excellent RCT evidence of effectiveness with benefit significantly greater than risk (Sever et al. 2004; Hippisley-Cox et al. 2007). Whether this is cost-effective will depend on therapy acquisition cost but generic statins remain cost-effective at these low-risk levels. However, substantially more individuals need treatment to prevent one event with high 'numbers-needed-to-treat' (NNTs). For individuals of moderate CVD risk (~10–20%/10yr) without significant contraindications, low-dose (10mg) simvastatin became the first long-term chronic treatment available for pharmacy purchase without a doctor's prescription, but where the National Health Service had decided not to fund.

The beliefs and wishes of the informed patient must be considered. Some individuals will wish to reduce relative risk even when their absolute risk is low. For others, even at higher risk, suggesting long-term medicine can be psychologically difficult to accept, converting them from 'a person into a patient' with awareness of morbidity and mortality. Individuals require full counselling about screening, and treatment benefits and risks.

12.7 How should we identify individuals at CVD risk?

Most management will occur in primary care where computerized records of individuals with existing CVD or diabetes will be known, and algorithms for recall and review will be in place.

Routine recording of tobacco use, blood pressure, and lipids allow automated computer algorithms to calculate a patient's approximate risk. Risk does not immediately recede as soon as blood pressure or cholesterol are treated and there is need to take account of family history. Where data are absent, computer programs could impute 'average' (or better 'likely') values for that patient to identify individuals to be called for CVD screening. Risk factors can then be measured and the prior 'theoretical' risk updated to an actual calculation. After the first formal screening changes in risk with advancing age or new risk factors will automatically compute.

The classical algorithms for the assessment of coronary and cerebrovascular risk of Framingham (Anderson *et al.* 1991) (which followed 5,200 individuals for >40yrs with excellent prospective data collection and follow up) has stood the test of time. Disadvantages include older data before risk factor management, a USA population, and less applicable to modern European and UK populations. Any risk algorithm will only approximate to its own population and potentially less well to other populations, and may not fully adjust, for example, for ethnicity and deprivation. Individual risk prediction is much less precise than might be suggested by a population algorithm.

12.8 Risk calculation and treatment targets

It must be emphasized that when an individual has sufficient risk to require intervention, all contributory risk factors should be addressed. A blood pressure target can be set at <140/<90 (<130/<80 in diabetes). Similarly, a cholesterol target of <4mmol/L is suggested and for LDL-C <2mmol/L (The Joint British Societies 2005; National Institute for Health and Clinical Excellence 2007). The greater the

LDL-C reduction the greater the relative risk reduction, and benefit is seen at both high and low absolute risk. CVD risk commences at LDL-C values well below those present in almost all individuals, so a 'fire and forget' approach has been suggested that all at-risk individuals should receive a standard dose of a generic statin (simvastatin 40mg or pravastatin) with a significant outcome-evidence base. The low acquisition cost gives a much more beneficial cost–benefit analysis. 'Fire and forget' does not necessarily imply no further lipid measurements are needed, and neither does it mean that this will be an appropriate response to the highest risk individuals who are likely to need additional measures. Titration of statin dose, a more effective statin, or combination therapy may be appropriate in secondary prevention, FH or in highest-risk primary prevention patients.

Efforts have been made in Europe to develop a country-specific algorithm, the SCORE system, but as data are often missing for morbidity in the European studies it has had to be developed from mortality studies with adjustment for morbidity, and with different scores in different communities.

Recently, a general practice database has been interrogated to produce an UK-specific algorithm, QRisk (Hippisley-Cox *et al.* 2007, 2008a,b). It validates well within a separate cohort of the same population, and fairly well in a separate population. Records from millions of patients are a major strength, but incomplete data are a substantial weakness. QRisk imputes values for missing data but concern arises when around two thirds of values are missing for analytes such as HDL-C. Different, non-standardized measurement methods for blood pressure and lipids will be partly offset by data volume. Better identification of deprivation as a CVD risk that would be valuable, but classical risk factors may congregate and co-travel within deprived populations. If more values are imputed for classical risk factors, then their precision will reduce, and greater identification of deprivation as a CVD risk may be more apparent than real. As general practice data accumulate in embedded algorithms, better prediction in a 'continuous improvement' model will be welcomed.

CVD risk algorithms embedded in primary care databases will also require systems applicable outside the surgery and in secondary care. There is significant imprecision in any algorithm and a patient's risk assessed with one system will inevitably vary in another. For statins at least benefit exceeds risk well below a 20%/10yr threshold and an individual would benefit whether risk might be 15% or 25%. If different methods are in place, decisions to treat (or not treat) based on one system should be accepted even if another system gives a somewhat different outcome.

12.9 **What is the evidence of benefit from lipid-lowering?**

Dietary change, lifestyle modification, and various drug groups can all reduce this global risk, but it was the advent in 1989 of the well-tolerated statins that changed outlook. Many large long-term statin trials have been undertaken since the '4S' (Scandinavian Simvastatin Survival Study) trial (Scandinavian Simvastatin Survival Study Group 1994). Further studies (Downs et al. 1998; Heart Protection Study Collaborative Group 2002; Colhoun et al. 2004; Sever et al. 2004; Cholesterol Treatment Trialists' Collaborators 2005) have substantially extended the evidence base and the guidelines of the Joint British Societies have now been updated (The Joint British Societies 2005), and the 20%/10yr threshold has been endorsed by NICE (National Institute for Health and Clinical Excellence 2007; NICE GDG). The Cholesterol Treatment Trialists' Collaborators have examined the relationship between cholesterol lowering and cardiovascular disease risk in more than 90,000 patients in 14 randomized, placebo-controlled trials of statin treatment, and demonstrated a 23% decrease in CHD for each 1mmol/L reduction in LDL-C (Cholesterol Treatment Trialists' Collaborators 2005). This applied to men and women, primary or secondary CVD prevention, up to the age of 85yrs, in smokers and non-smokers, with high triglycerides or low HDL-C, and whether there was hypertension or diabetes.

Very similar data from this group are shown in 18,686 individuals with diabetes (Cholesterol Treatment Trialists' Collaborators 2008). Five years after the diagnosis of diabetes, individuals have a risk for a first CVD event as great as that of a non-diabetic individual with a previous heart attack. CVD risk is also increased around twofold in individuals with impaired glucose tolerance before the development of diabetes. In the Heart Protection Study (Heart Protection Study Collaborative Group 2002) of 20,000 individuals, the 30% who had diabetes were at higher absolute risk and had the same relative benefit both in coronary disease and stroke reduction. In a primary prevention study in type 2 diabetes (CARDS) (Colhoun 2004), 10mg atorvastatin reduced CVD risk 37%, with a 36% (9–55% CI) reduction in CHD and a 48% (11–69%) reduction in stroke.

Figure 12.1 shows the rates of CVD plotted against the LDL-C concentrations in primary and secondary CVD prevention studies with statins (and colestyramine) for placebo and treated populations, or for lower and higher intensity of treatment. Lower CVD occurred with lower achieved LDL-C concentrations to LDL levels below 2mmol/L.

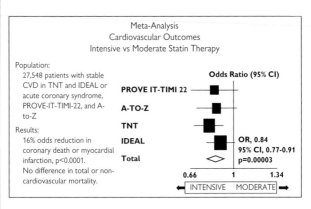

Figure 12.1 The relationship between the rates of major cardiac events and LDL-cholesterol concentrations (mmol/L) in various statin* primary and secondary prevention cardiovascular outcome trials

Points on the right-hand end of each line represent placebo-treated populations connected on the left-hand end with actively treated populations, or represent lower intensity treated populations with higher intensity treated populations.

* The LRC-CPPT study was a colestyramine and not a statin study.

Source: The Joint British Societies (British Cardiac Society, British Hypertension Society, Diabetes UK, HEART UK, Primary Care Cardiovascular Society, Stroke Association) (2005). *Heart*, **91**, V1–52.

12.10 **Starting lipid-lowering drug therapy**

Patients presenting with acute CVD should have a statin started immediately with random cholesterol measurement. A fasting profile should be measured at subsequent specialist or primary care follow up to ensure that targets are achieved and to assess fasting triglycerides. In primary prevention asymptomatic patients, and in patients with known stable CVD, two separate lipid measurements (one as a fasting profile) should be assessed before treatment. Secondary causes of dyslipidaemia (such as hypothyroidism, uncontrolled diabetes, excess alcohol, obesity, certain drugs) should be addressed. The initial statin treatment should be one with CVD outcome evidence and a low acquisition cost. Lipid modifying effects will be fully evident a month after initiation. If individuals have entirely normal triglyceride values, then subsequent cholesterol monitoring can be non-fasting, but if there is significant hypertriglyceridaemia then fasting profiles will be needed.

First choice statin is determined largely by cost, for simvastatin and pravastatin are off patent, and costs have fallen to about 15% of the original value, before moving to alternatives. Most of a statin's effect is obtained with the entry low dose. About 6% extra LDL-C-lowering is seen with each dose doubling. At a given mg dose of a statin, there is a further approximate 6% LDL-C-lowering moving from pravastatin or fluvastatin to simvastatin, a further 6% to atorvastatin, and 8–9% further again moving to rosuvastatin. Low-dose (10mg) simvastatin can be purchased from a pharmacist without a doctor's prescription for suitable middle-older age individuals with sufficient risk (10–20% CVD/10yr risk).

Patients with severe or poorly responsive dyslipidaemia should be referred for specialist advice. Where there is significant mixed dyslipidaemia, or hypertriglyceridaemia, persisting after LDL-C has reached target in high-risk patients, additional therapy with a fibrate, nicotinic acid, or omega-3 fish oils can be considered, and again specialist advice may be appropriate but would not be routine.

Patients at very high risk, and those with very high cholesterol (and LDL cholesterol) levels can require additional treatment. Bile acid sequestrant agents (such as colestyramine) with some CVD outcome evidence have been used for decades but are not easy to take or tolerate. More recently, a specific inhibitor of cholesterol transport across the enterocyte, ezetimibe, has become available which will lower LDL-C by ~18–25% added to other treatments. It is well tolerated with low side effects, but as yet has no CVD outcome data. FH patients are almost always going to require combination therapy. Ezetimibe is useful for individuals with previous statin myositis or intolerance.

12.11 **Statin safety**

Statin use is very safe, with death, serious or persistent (after treatment cessation) side effects being rare. Moderate side effects, classically of muscle discomfort, are perceived by a significant number of individuals even without a rise in creatine kinase and may limit therapy. A different statin or a lower dose may be appropriate. Creatine kinase is not a useful routine measurement in an asymptomatic patient as it may rise significantly after even modest, usual day-to-day exercise. It should be recognized that statin safety exceeds that of low dose (75–150mg) aspirin by at least 10-fold, with greater relative gain.

Statin therapy has been very successful with a very low rate of serious side effects (Ballantyne et al. 2003). Severe myositis and rhabdomyolysis occurs approximately once in 30–50,000 patient-years of treatment. Patients should be warned that if they get generalized muscle discomfort, pain, tenderness, or weakness lasting more than a couple of days that they should have creatine kinase checked, and consideration given to at least temporarily stopping the statin, although very rarely will the symptoms be drug related. In side effect terms, there is little to choose between the five statins available, with published CVD outcome data for four (atorvastatin, fluvastatin, pravastatin, simvastatin), while for rosuvastatin the JUPITER study is announced as positive. Many drugs are metabolized through the cytochrome P450 3A4 pathway, as are simvastatin and atorvastatin. Fluvastatin, pravastatin, and rosuvastatin are metabolized via different routes and may therefore pose some less risk of drug interactions, for example, in patients taking drugs such as ciclosporin or antiretrovirals.

In FH, in some patients with diabetes, and in individuals with very premature CVD statins will be required in younger women. Women of child-bearing age should be advised to stop statin therapy from conception planning until the end of breast-feeding.

12.12 **How low to go?—cholesterol or LDL-C or non-HDL-C**

Questions remain as to whether all patients at sufficient risk should have a fixed effective statin dose, whether the aim should be a sufficient fall in LDL-C, whether there should be a target or targets to achieve, or whether the largest fall sensibly possible should be achieved. The epidemiological data, and substantially the intervention data also, suggest that there is a linear relationship between the degree of LDL-C-lowering and the extent of reduction in CVD achieved, and this is true to quite low levels of LDL-C. Almost all individuals in adulthood have LDL-C levels above those of ≤1mmol/L seen in neonates. Recent studies comparing standard statin treatments with more intensive statin treatments have shown trends or significant reductions in CVD risk (depending on the particular study, its size, and duration) with the higher dose regimens, the extra reduction in risk being related to the degree of difference in LDL-C between the groups, at least to LDL-C levels of 1.7mmol/L (Cannon et al. 2004; La Rosa et al. 2005). Such gains need to be offset by the modest but present risk of a higher side effect profile.

While different final LDL-C levels were achieved between the groups in these studies, none of them had a planned treat-to-target regimen. Nonetheless, targets have been set in a number of guidelines. The targets for LDL-C in the United States are set at different levels depending on the potential risk of different patient groups, in primary or secondary prevention down to <1.7mmol/L. In the United Kingdom, a simpler approach has been taken of a single target for LDL-C of <2mmol/L for all patients at sufficient risk to require lipid-lowering treatment. Targets are to an extent arbitrary, but are useful in management and audit. They allow a more straightforward approach and facilitate audit of achievements, but in its application it should be recognized that it may not be appropriate or possible to reach such a target in all patients. Thus, if desirable targets for cholesterol and

LDL-C of <4mmol/L and <2mmol/L, respectively, are considered, then one may then set a reasonably high percentage standards for audit criteria of the number of patients achieving values <5mmol/L and <3mmol/L, respectively. However, it is insufficient to reach LDL-C <3mmol/L in a very high-risk patient if their initial value was only just >3mmol/L. It should be possible for the great majority of statin-treated patients to achieve an LDL-C reduction of ≥30%.

12.13 Hypertriglyceridaemia assessment and management

While indications for LDL-C lowering with statins for CVD prevention are clear, management of individuals with significant mixed dyslipidaemia or with severe hypertriglyceridaemia is more problematical. It is essential in such individuals to seek for, and to manage, associated disorders contributing to the abnormal lipid profile. Hypothyroidism, abnormal hepatic or renal function, diabetes, alcohol excess, and obesity may all be significant players.

In individuals with more moderate hypertriglyceridaemia the CVD risk is increased, especially if HDL-C is low. First-line management is still to lower LDL-C with a statin. Where residual hypertriglyceridaemia persists in very high-risk individuals (such as with type 2 diabetes), clinical judgement will be needed about combination statin–fibrate treatment. Gemfibrozil should not be used with a statin because of a very much higher adverse event rate. Fenofibrate would usually be the fibrate of choice. The recent FIELD study in 10,000 patients with type 2 diabetes provided some limited CVD outcome evidence (Keech et al. 2005).

With severe hypertriglyceridaemia (>10mmol/L and especially >20mmol/L), pancreatitis can result even in the absence of other causes. Individuals who are obese, diabetic, or have taken excess alcohol are at high risk, usually in the context of an underlying mixed dyslipidaemia. Management in the acute situation is calorie restriction and intravenous fluids, and the triglycerides will tend to settle substantially over 2–4 days. Statins are not of value in this situation of severe hypertriglyceridaemia. Fibrates may be appropriate, as may be concentrated omega-3 triglycerides (such as Omacor® 3–4g daily rather than the 1–2g daily licensed for CHD prevention), while insulin therapy may be helpful in glucose-intolerant patients.

References

Anderson KM, Odell PM, Wilson PW, and Kannel WB (1991). Cardiovascular disease risk profiles: the Framingham study. *American Heart Journal*, **121**, 293–8.

Ballantyne CM, Corsini A, Davidson MH, *et al.* (2003). Risk for myopathy with statin therapy in high-risk patients: expert panel review. *Archives of Internal Medicine*, **163**, 553–64.

Cannon CP, Braunwald E, McCabe CH, *et al.* for the TIMI-22 investigators (2004). Pravastatin or atorvastatin evaluation and infection therapy— Thrombolysis In Myocardial Infarction 22 (TIMI-22) investigators. Intensive versus moderate lipid lowering with statins after acute coronary syndromes. *The New England Journal of Medicine*, **350**, 1495–504.

Cholesterol Treatment Trialists' Collaborators (2005). Efficacy and safety of cholesterol-lowering treatment: prospective meta-analysis of data from 90,056 participants in 14 randomised trials of statins. *The Lancet*, **366**, 1267–78.

Cholesterol Treatment Trialists' Collaborators (2008). Efficacy of cholesterol-lowering treatment in 18,686 people with diabetes in 14 randomised trials of statins: a meta-analysis. *The Lancet*, **371**, 117–25.

Colhoun HM, Betteridge DJ, Durrington PN, *et al.* on behalf of the CARDS investigators (2004). Primary prevention of cardiovascular disease with atorvastatin in type 2 diabetes in the Collaborative Atorvastatin Diabetes Study (CARDS): a multicentre, randomised, placebo-controlled trial. *The Lancet*, **364**, 685–96.

Downs JR, Clearfield M, Weis S, *et al.* for the AFCAPS/TexCAPS Research Group (1998). Primary prevention of acute coronary events with lovastatin in men and women with average cholesterol levels: results of AFCAPS/TexCAPS. Air Force/Texas Coronary Atherosclerosis Prevention Study. *JAMA*, **279**, 1615–22.

Heart Protection Study Collaborative Group (2002). MRC/BHF Heart Protection Study of cholesterol lowering with simvastatin in 20,536 high-risk individuals: a randomised placebo-controlled trial. *The Lancet*, **360**, 7–22.

Hippisley-Cox J, Coupland C, Vinogradova Y, Robson J, May M, and Brindle P (2007). Derivation and validation of QRISK, a new cardiovascular risk score for the United Kingdom: prospective open cohort study. *British Medical Journal*, **335**, 136.

Hippisley-Cox J, Coupland C, Vinogradova Y, Robson J, May M, and Brindle P (2008a). The performance of the QRISK cardiovascular prediction algorithm in an external sample of patients from General Practice: a validation study. *Heart*, **94**, 34–9.

Hippisley-Cox J, Coupland C, Vinogradova Y, *et al.* (2008b). Predicting cardiovascular risk in England and Wales: prospective derivation and validation of QRISK2. *British Medical Journal*, **336**, 1457–82.

Keech A, Simes RJ, Barter P, *et al.* and the FIELD Study Investigators (2005). Effects of long-term fenofibrate therapy on cardiovascular events in 9795 people with type 2 diabetes (the FIELD study— Fenofibrate Intervention and Event Lowering in Diabetes study): randomised controlled trial. *The Lancet*, **366**, 1849–61.

La Rosa JC, Grundy SM, Waters DD, *et al.* for the Treating to New Targets (TNT) investigators (2005). Intensive lipid lowering with atorvastatin in patients with stable coronary disease. *The New England Journal of Medicine*, **352**, 1425–35.

Marks D, Thorogood M, Neil HA, *et al.* (2003). A review on the diagnosis, natural history, and treatment of familial hypercholesterolaemia. *Atherosclerosis*, **168**, 1–14.

National Institute for Health and Clinical Excellence (2007a). Statins for the prevention of cardiovascular events. NICE Technology Appraisal 94.

National Institute for Health and Clinical Excellence (2007b). Ezetimibe for the treatment of primary (heterozygous-familial and non-familial) hypercholesterolaemia. NICE, London, Technology Appraisal 132.

Scandinavian Simvastatin Survival Study Group (1994). Randomised trial of cholesterol lowering in 4,444 patients with coronary heart disease: the Scandinavian Simvastatin Survival Study (4S). *The Lancet*, **344**, 1383–9.

Sever PS, Dahlof B, Poulter N, *et al.* for the ASCOT investigators (2004). Prevention of coronary and stroke events with atorvastatin in hypertensive patients with average or lower than average cholesterol concentrations, in the Anglo-Scandinavian Cardiac Outcomes Trial—Lipid Lowering Arm (ASCOT-LLA): a multicentre randomised controlled trial. *The Lancet*, **361**, 1149–58.

Scientific Steering Committee on behalf of the Simon Broome Register Group (1999). Mortality in treated heterozygous familial hypercholesterolaemia: implications for clinical management. *Atherosclerosis*, **142**, 105–12.

The Joint British Societies (British Cardiac Society, British Hypertension Society, Diabetes UK, HEART UK, Primary Care Cardiovascular Society, Stroke Association) (2005). Joint British Societies' Second Guidelines for the prevention of cardiovascular disease in clinical practice. *Heart*, **91**, V1–52.

Index